REINVENTING THE SEXES

Race, Gender, and Science

Anne Fausto-Sterling, General Editor

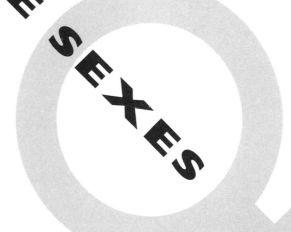

MARIANNE VAN DEN WIJNGAARD

REINVENTING THE SEXES

*The Biomedical Construction
of Femininity and
Masculinity*

Indiana University Press
Bloomington • Indianapolis

Manufactured in the United States of America

Library of Congress Cataloging-in-Publication Data

Wijngaard, Marianne van den.
Reinventing the sexes : the biomedical construction of femininity and masculinity /
Marianne van den Wijngaard.
    p.   cm. — (Race, gender, and science)
Previously published: Amsterdam, Netherlands : Uitgeverij Eburon, 1991.
Includes bibliographical references and index.
ISBN 0–253–33250–8 (alk. paper). — ISBN 0–253–21087–9 (pbk. : alk. paper)
1. Sex differences—Research—History. I. Title. II. Series.
QP81.5.W55 1997
612.6–dc20   96-41378
1   2   3   4   5   02   01   00   99   98   97

WE CALL CONTRARY TO
NATURE WHAT HAPPENS
CONTRARY TO CUSTOM;
NOTHING IS ANYTHING
BUT ACCORDING TO
NATURE, WHATEVER IT
MAY BE.
LET THIS UNIVERSAL AND
NATURAL REASON DRIVE
OUT OF US THE ERROR
AND ASTONISHMENT THAT
NOVELTY BRINGS US.

MICHEL DE MONTAIGNE

CONTENTS

PREFACE

This book unravels the role of biomedical knowledge about masculinity and femininity in attributing meaning to physical appearance. Without the resistance of some scientists in the field of behavioral neuroendocrinology to my research findings, this book would probably never have been written. Their objections proved that the political connotations of my work exceeded my expectations and thus made it more important to publish my results.

On the other hand, many individuals and institutions have supported my research and writing, and I wish to express my appreciation and gratitude here. Financial support came from the Belle van Zuylen Institute, the Faculty of Biology, and the Faculty of Psychology at the University of Amsterdam. I received very valuable inspiration, ideas, and support from Lynda Birke, the late Ruth Bleier, Rosi Braidotti, Christien Brinkgreve, Jaqueline Cramer, Walter Everaerd, Anne Fausto-Sterling, Joke 't Hart, Francien de Jonge, Evelyn Fox Keller, Ruth Hubbard, Chunglin Kwa, Gloria Meredith, Fernando Lopez da Sylva, Annemarie Mol, Nanne van der Poll, Koos Slob, Pieter van der Schoot, and Jan Wattel.

I also wish to express my gratitude to the members of the research network for Women's Studies in Biology and Medicine: Els Branssen, Christien Brouwer, Lidy Schoon, and Ineke van Wingerden. Special thanks go to my most inspiring colleague and friend, Nelly Oudshoorn. Adele Clarke and Anne Fausto-Sterling offered wonderful suggestions for completing the manuscript.

I wish to thank Polly Rademaker and Dini Winthagen for their efficiency in providing materials from the library of the Faculty of Biology and from other libraries. I am grateful to have found Lee Mitzman, who supported me both in professionally polishing my Dutch English to make the contents of this book shine and in helping me think of approaches to problems during the final preparations for publication.

Finally, I would like to express my gratitude to my family and friends. Although my parents died long before I completed the manuscript, I would like to share the joy of publishing it with them. My mother always encouraged me to start projects that interested me and, equally importantly, to finish them. My father motivated me to investigate this subject and taught me to enjoy everything life has to offer, even in difficult times. These abilities proved indispensable in the periods of doubt and uncertainty that accompanied the research and writing involved in this book.

I want to thank my friends who have supported me through life in general and in particular while I was writing this book: Jaqueline Hoekstra and Tine Veldkamp. They shared the fascination of seeing the world through women's eyes, each with her own degree of radicalism and means of expression. I learned from their strategies for coping with difficult situations. Equally valuable was the support of my male friends: Ward, Hans, and Jan. They showed me that men benefit as much as women from feminist practice, which strives to do justice to all.

Some of these chapters have been published previously. Chapter 2 was published in the *Journal of the History of Biology,* vol. 24, no. 1 (1991): 19–49. Chapter 3 was also published in the *Journal of the History of Biology,* vol. 27, no. 1 (1994): 61–90. An earlier version of chapter 4 appeared in *Kennis en Methode,* vol. 13, no. 4 (1989): 382–96, and a Norwegian translation appeared in *Nytt om Kvinneforskning,* vol. 14, no. 4 (1990): 35–46.

FEMININITY AND WOMEN IN BIOLOGY AND FEMINIST THEORY

Gender Trouble and Making Sex

This book reveals how biomedical scientists reinvented the sexes and how they assigned new and different meanings to gender, masculinity, and femininity in their investigation of the effects of sex hormones. The words "sex" and "gender" that appear in this sentence acquired connected and interwoven meanings in the biomedical research concerned. Thus, the study provides an excellent opportunity for reconsidering the theoretical division between sex and gender. At the beginning of the 1980s this division came under increasing question. At that time the feminist biologists Ruth Bleier, Ruth Hubbard, Anne Fausto-Sterling, and many others began questioning sex, or rather knowledge about sex, in current and past biomedical research.[1] Their work meant that feminist scholars saw scientific discourses about sex no longer as mere representations of nature, or as facts resulting from value-free investigations; scholars recognized that the results of scientific experiments were subject to sociocultural interpretations and assessments in which women traditionally had little impact compared to men. Gradually, it became conceivable that sex was not as universal or ahistorical as scientists had previously led us to believe; sex turned out to be more culturally determined than scientists had initially imagined. In her book *Gender Trouble*, feminist philosopher Judith Butler wonders: "Are the ostensibly natural facts of sex discursively produced by various scientific discourses in the service of other political and social interests? If the immutable character of sex is contested, perhaps this construct called 'sex' is as culturally constructed as gender; indeed, perhaps it was always already gender, with the consequence that the distinction between sex and gender turns out to be no distinction at all."[2] In *Making Sex,* Thomas Laqueur argues that "almost everything one wants to say about sex—however sex is understood—already has in it a claim about gender."[3] He uses historical analysis of scientific texts and anatomical drawings of female and male genitals to demonstrate the ways culture suffuses and changes representations of the human body. The chronological span of his examination ends with the work of Freud at the turn of the century.

Laqueur's historical findings are repeated in the development of recent biological knowledge and current medical practice. He distinguishes two models in historical anatomical drawings and scientific texts (the one-sex model and the two-sex model) and explains that female organs were represented as a lesser form of male organs in accordance with the pre-Enlightenment view that woman was a lesser variant of man. During the period that the one-sex model was dominant, scientists considered female anatomy an imperfect version of male anatomy. The vagina was viewed as an interior penis, the womb as a scrotum, and the ovaries as testicles. In the pre-Enlightenment period, sex or the body was to be understood as an epiphenomenon, while gender, which is currently perceived as a cultural category, was considered primary or "real." Especially before the seventeenth century, Laqueur argues, "sex was a sociological and not an ontological category." Thus, "the body is a representation, not the foundation of gender."[4] This outlook changed in the eighteenth century, when the two-sex model arose. Although this shift was neither ubiquitous, simultaneous, nor permanent, the one-sex model was confronted with a powerful alternative. At that time, male and female sex organs, which had previously shared the same names (e.g., ovaries and testicles) acquired linguistic distinctions. The two-sex model assigned names to organs that had not had individual labels according to the one-sex model, such as the vagina. Since the beginning of the two-sex model, the two sexes have been considered binary opposites with incommensurable organs, functions, and sensations.[5] Moreover, the rise of the two-sex model coincided with a sharpening of the division between body and spirit; the body became the foundation for gender. Laqueur stresses that statements made within both the one-sex model and the two-sex model are burdened with the cultural views of women and men. "Two incommensurable sexes were, and are, as much the products of culture as was, and is, the one-sex model."[6] In Laqueur's two-sex model, sex replaces our idea of gender as a primary foundational category. The new framework distinguished natural concepts from social ones. This book outlines the cycle of historical repetition. We will see how between 1959 and 1985 the one-sex model was replaced by a two-sex model or what we may consider a multi-sex model. As in Laqueur's study, we will see how the division between the natural and the social became problematic with the rise of a two-sex model in the 1970s. We will also see how the conceptual division between masculinity and femininity has caused difficulties in scientists' recent biological research. All in all we may wonder to what extent the theoretically strict dividing line between the social and the natural, as well as between masculinity and femininity and even male and female, is a cultural artifact.

If we simply look at the facts as they are, a universal dividing line even between the sexes never existed in nature. Anne Fausto-Sterling proposes to distinguish five sexes instead of two, in order to make it possible for people with ambiguous sex to live a more human life.[7] Intersex babies are born more often than most of us know. A reliable number is hard to come by, but Fausto-Sterling takes 1.7 percent of all births as an order of magnitude. She scoured the medical literature for frequency estimates of different types of intersexuality.

People with physical characteristics from both sexes have always been among us. Throughout history, they have been viewed as problematic creatures, not because they were ill, but because their ambiguous bodies inevitably challenged the boundaries of sex and gender. Medical practitioners classified such individuals as pseudohermaphrodites and consulted on deciding their fate. Their task consisted of advising judicial officials. Sometimes ecclesiastical authorities also became involved.[8]

Thus, even nature is less than scrupulous in creating two distinct sexes. People born as intersex individuals violated the moral laws of sexuality in Western societies and therefore often entered the sphere of medical intervention. In his introduction to *Herculine Barbin: Being the Recently Discovered Memoirs of a Nineteenth-Century French Hermaphrodite,* and in *The History of Sexuality,* Michel Foucault suggests that the category of sex is constructed according to a historically specific mode of sexuality.[9] Normally, sex, in its capacity as female or male, is postulated as the "cause" of sexual experience, behavior, and desire. Judith Butler argues, however, that this ostensible "cause" might just as well be regarded as an "effect."[10] This situation seems to have been true for Herculine Barbin, who was raised as a girl until doctors in the nineteenth century discovered she was actually a pseudohermaphrodite with characteristics of both sexes. Herculine Barbin was raised in a world with only women and developed a sexual relationship with one of the girls. Her desire for a girl caused a scandal and resulted in her being classified as a man by officials. While her ambiguous body was viewed as a medical curiosity, it was not considered the most urgent problem; her sexual desire for girls, seen as a man's desire, was regarded as incompatible with her body and environment. She had to leave the girls' school and her village. Her official sex and name were changed; after the intervention, Herculine was called Camille or Abel. These names mirror the instability of this individual's identity, which ended in despondency and suicide. The story of Herculine shows how desire shaped sex at a time when both aspects were expected to form a heterosexual unity. Perhaps "desire" is the only "real" thing, as "male" and "female" are certainly not universal natural categories.

In the nineteenth century, officials tried to adapt Herculine's desire to the moral laws while leaving her body as it was. In the twentieth century, the bodies of pseudohermaphrodites have been surgically shaped into one sex or the other. Modern medical practice and surgery in particular have become increasingly adept at regulating the relationship of bodies to themselves and to each other, as Stefan Hirschauer elegantly demonstrates. He argues that the anatomical body is an accomplishment of the sculptural practice of operations, especially considering sex.[11] Moreover, psychologists assist pseudohermaphrodites as well as transsexuals in becoming truly feminine or masculine in psychological respects. This approach creates nonexistent natural categories of male/female and masculine/feminine with the help of scientists, doctors, and psychologists. Nowadays, it seems easier to transform sex than to change gender.

Until recently, however, gender was considered the changeable characteristic. In this study, I will demonstrate how sex and gender have been reinvented during an era in which masculinity and femininity are no longer taken for granted. To this end, I have chosen the production of knowledge in neuroendocrinology of behavior and focus on the body of knowledge about the differentiation of the brain into male or female traits and the consequences for feminine or masculine behavior.

The story begins in 1959, when sex roles and the position of women and of men were hardly questioned, and continues throughout the 1960s, the 1970s, and the 1980s. The production of this knowledge became significant during the late 1960s, when sex roles and sex differences in the social positions of women and men ceased to be self-evident. Soon, researchers in disciplines such as sociology, anthropology, psychology, and biology began to raise similar questions about sex differences and their origins. Most feminists subscribed to the thesis of Simone de Beauvoir, who argued that "women are not born, but made to be women," suggesting that only sociocultural factors affect the development of femininity in behavior.[12] This thesis was contradicted by knowledge developed through biomedical research. Since 1959, biomedical researchers have described how the sexual organs bathe the embryo with hormones in the womb, resulting in the birth of an individual with a male or a female brain.[13] This idea underlies the *organization theory,* which was postulated in that year. Scientists identified a distinctively male or female brain to predict future behavioral development in a masculine or feminine direction. Over the past thirty years, they have increasingly claimed that types of behavior in males and females, both animal and human, are affected by prenatal hormones. In humans, such behavior varies from sexual orientation, career choice or mothering, to mathematical and verbal skills.[14] Most effects of hormones on differentiating brains turned out to be categorically divided according to traditional perceptions of feminine and masculine characteristics: Male hormones potentiated future behavior; female hormones potentiated future male behavior.

This story is about one strand of the nature versus nurture debates, the struggles over difference that persist under old and new rubrics and through old and new vocabularies. To simplify the positions: Feminists, on the one hand, have localized the origins of all sex differences in behavior, in social structures, and in education. Biomedical scientists, on the other hand, basing their arguments on biological knowledge about the hormonal effects on prenatal brain development, have argued that differences in feminine and masculine behavior are also likely to depend on biological distinctions between women and men. Be that as it may, many people have assumed that genetic differences underlay the different positions of women and men in society, thus localizing the origin of disparate behavior between the sexes in individual women and men. Some journalists, popularizing biological knowledge, have even warned that the social changes demanded by feminism will harm human nature.[15]

Although the consequences of these positions are politically contradictory, many feminists and biomedical researchers have shared their interest in the subject of sex differences since the late 1960s. Especially sex differences in behavior have become a very popular subject of biomedical research (fig 1.1). Until the late 1970s, however, most feminists ignored the results of biological investigations into sex differences. Some rationalized their fear of ideologically incorrect science by arguing that biology is not the right discipline for producing knowledge about human behavior.[16]

This story is not about determining who is right or wrong. The questions are: How have biomedical scientists constructed images of femininity and masculinity? How has feminism contributed to changes in or persistence of these images?

To convey the magnitude of the constructing power of laboratory investigations in general and especially with regard to masculinity and femininity, I will compare the influence of anthropologist Margaret Mead (who suggested that nurture was the most important element in behavioral development) on general perceptions of masculinity and femininity during the 1930s with recent laboratory studies concerning the impact of nature on the development of sex differences in behavior.

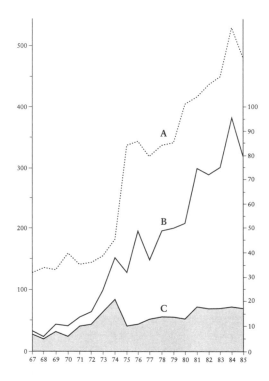

Fig. 1.1. Research on sex differences published between 1967 and 1985. (Titles retrieved from Biomedical Datalog.)
A = Titles on sex differences in general; number of articles on left vertical axis.
B = Titles on sex differences in brain development; number of articles on right vertical axis.
C = Relative contribution B/A in percent on right vertical axis.

Back and Forth between Nurture and Nature

By the 1970s, both the issue of whether nurture or nature underlay masculinity and femininity in behavior and the opposition to the nature claim had become familiar issues. Moreover, it was not the first time that disciplinary competence in this matter was questioned. In the 1930s, Margaret Mead's investigations of human temperament in non-Western societies had increased the influence of anthropology and sociology on the production of knowledge about human behavior. Mead argued that western conceptions of masculinity or femininity in behavior could vary considerably from non-Western images of the sexes. She studied the temperaments of women and men in three societies: the Arapesh, where the ideal consists of mildly responsive men and women; the Mundugumor, where the ideal prescribes violent, aggressive men and women; and the Tchambuli, where the ideal involves dominant women and dependent men.[17] Mead concluded:

> If those temperamental attitudes which we have traditionally regarded as feminine can so easily be set up as the masculine pattern in one tribe, and in another be outlawed for the majority of women as well as for the majority of men, we no longer have any basis for regarding such aspects of behavior as sex-linked.[18]

Mead alleged that while both aggressive and passive human dispositions exist, designating such behavior as universally masculine and feminine would be illegitimate. She suggested that human nature was almost unbelievably malleable. According to Mead, "Standardized personality differences between the sexes are of this order, cultural creations to which each generation, male and female is trained to conform."[19]

In 1928 Mead published *Coming of Age in Samoa;* in this book she reported on her investigations of adolescent girls in Samoa during 1925.[20] She considered intercultural comparison the ideal method to obtain insight into the differential effects of cultural expectations and the effects of biological changes during adolescence. Mead concluded that growing up in Samoa is much easier than in the United States because of the general casualness of Samoan society: "For Samoa is a place where no one plays for very high stakes, no one suffers for his conditions or fights to the death for special ends."[21] Mead saw the difficulties of people during adolescence in the Western world as a consequence of a culture with many and conflicting demands, double standards about sexuality, and so forth, rather than as caused by bodily changes as most scientists believed. Mead's work was popular and widely read. An important reason for its notoriety was the criticism of her nonconventional findings.[22]

The most well-known objections to Mead's work came from the Australian anthropologist D. Freeman. He also conducted field studies in Samoa and reported on them in *Mead and Samoa: The Making and Unmaking of an Anthropological Myth.*[23] He started his investigations on Samoa in the 1940s and continued in the 1960s in the German part of

Samoa, although Mead studied girls in the American part of Samoa. Mead's *Coming of Age* is not a general ethnography of Samoa; it is a systematic study guided by a particular question. Freeman's guiding principle was the rejection of Mead's claims; Mead rather than Samoa was the subject of his line of argument. Where Mead describes Samoan culture as flexible, Freeman shows how rigid it is. Where Mead says that war has an almost ceremonial character, Freeman tells about bloody battles and the extinction of complete villages. Where Mead pictures an image of a carefree sex life, Freeman stresses an almost Victorian morality. Where Mead speaks about a harmonious adolescence, Freeman cites data of teenage criminality comparable to those of Chicago. Freeman's rejection is complete; none of Mead's claims goes unopposed. This led to doubts about the validity of Freeman's work, although Samoan culture is not a monolithic entity and the German part of Samoa can be quite different from the American part. Freeman suggested that Mead's work was the result of *cultural determinism,* meaning that biological factors are irrelevant to an understanding of human behavior.[24] Freeman began a correspondence with Mead in 1964 about his study. However, he sent her the complete manuscript, as it was published in 1983, only a few months before Mead died in 1978. Remarkably enough Freeman did not mention Mead's comments. We may wonder why, and also why he waited so long to publish his book. Was he afraid of Mead, or can we think of other reasons?

Although Freeman did not explicitly refer to sociobiology, in his writing he was clearly charmed by the idea of a genetic basis for human behavior; his book was positively received by the famous ethologists N. Tinbergen and I. Eibl Eibesfeldt. During the 1960s and early 1970s scientific publications with this tenor were not appreciated. The memory of World War II and the Nazi application of eugenic principles and practices was too fresh.[25] During the late 1970s books referring to a genetic basis for human behavior clearly could again be published, as witness *The Selfish Gene* by R. Dawkins (1976) and *On Human Nature* by E. O. Wilson (1978). These books countered ideas about the effects of nurture as proposed by feminist authors. By 1983 Freeman could be sure to gain appreciation and support for his work. This story illustrates how science always has political and ideological implications and how we can understand the popularity of a scientific explanation, either nature or nurture, within a cultural context.

Despite, or perhaps as a result of the criticism of Mead's work, the authority of anthropology and sociology in generating knowledge about human behavior was significantly strengthened. In the 1970s, Mead's work served as an inspiration to feminist scholars developing theories about the effect of nurture on behavior.

Unlike the view in the 1930s, however, current laboratory investigations of biological sex differences in human behavior are considered more scientific than are explorations of environmental variables.[26] In addition, science "works" by way of practices based on the knowledge it generates. To indicate how experimental research can change images and practices concerning masculinity and femininity, I will draw a parallel between a comparable case study on laboratory research and the present one.

In his article "Give Me a Laboratory and I Will Raise the World," Bruno Latour, an anthropologist of science, demonstrated the magnitude of the changes in scientific and social practice following Pasteur's laboratory research on anthrax. Latour described two sorts of changes. First, perceptions changed regarding anthrax as a disease. Before Pasteur's investigations, farmers and scientists regarded anthrax as a local phenomenon; they associated prevention and eradication of anthrax with local variables. Soil, wind, weather, animals, and even laborers were considered responsible for the incidence of the disease. Pasteur's findings changed this view. Instead of attributing anthrax to unpredictable local variables, Pasteur established that the disease resulted from a well-described cause: the microbe. Anthrax was a predictable outcome of infection by this microbe.

Second, methods to combat anthrax changed along with the image of the disease. We might claim that society was remodeled on the basis of laboratory practices: Microscale laboratory arrangements were applied on a larger scale in society. Before Pasteur's investigations, hygiene and vaccination were unknown weapons against anthrax. Latour generalized his conclusions as follows: "I claim that laboratories are among the few places where the very content of the trials made (within the walls of the laboratory) can alter the position of society, . . . where society and politics are renewed and transformed."[27]

Replacing the words "anthrax" and "microbes" with "sex differences" and "hormones" enables us to visualize the impact of this type of research on images of masculinity and femininity.

Comparable to the impact of Pasteur's investigations on thought and practices concerning anthrax, but unlike the effect of Mead's research on non-Western societies, knowledge based on the organization theory produced in laboratories is applied in medical treatment of pseudo-hermaphrodites. These individuals' ambiguous genitals are often attributed to abnormal hormone levels before birth. Questions arose as to the effect of these hormones on the differentiations within their brains and consequently on their behavior as well. About a decade after the initial proposal of the organization theory (1959), the behavior of a group of pseudohermaphrodites was studied. Indeed, the psychologists J. Money and A. Ehrhardt succeeded in confirming their hypothesis that prenatal hormones affected future feminine or masculine behavior among pseudo-hermaphrodites.[28]

As a consequence of Money and Ehrhardt's findings, physicians and psychiatrists involved in the medical treatment of pseudohermaphrodites in the 1970s supplemented surgical correction of the genitals with psychological counseling for becoming a "normal" woman or man.

Thus, physicians and psychiatrists joined biomedical scientists in their involvement in the construction of females and males as well as in that of femininity and masculinity. To formulate the questions raised by this story more precisely: How did scientists, physicians, and psychiatrists construct images of biological femininity and masculinity based on the organization theory? In which ways did feminism contribute to change or continuity of these images?

I will answer these questions by describing the subjects and dates of these investigations, as well as the individuals responsible for and the reasons behind the research conducted between 1959 and 1985 on the effects of hormones on male and female brain development and their consequences for masculine or feminine behavior. From my perspective, scientific facts do not emerge from the observation of results of experiments by individual scientists but are established in the interactions between different groups of people interested in a particular subject. These interactions can be characterized as negotiations, as they often involve more than mere acceptance of knowledge. A scientist's reputation can play a role, for example, in the acceptance of this person's findings by other scientists. Conversely, opportunities for publishing articles in scientific journals and for gaining acceptance of results affect scientists' professional reputations.

Groups of scientists sharing a special interest in knowledge about a subject form a network. Interactive processes in the network of people inside as well as outside laboratories determine the criteria for establishing scientific facts and the basis for accepting or rejecting information as knowledge. In our context, the professional groups (one individual may belong to several groups) involved in the production of knowledge about the development of feminine or masculine behavior include biomedical scientists from different disciplines, physicians, psychiatrists, journalists popularizing biomedical knowledge, psychologists, sociologists, and feminists of different "vintages." All these groups were and continue to be interested in the origins of sex differences in behavior, and they form a network for interaction concerning criteria for accepting or rejecting knowledge. In this analysis, groups of scientists or individuals engage in interaction about the acceptance of knowledge. The possibilities for groups of scientists or individuals to realize their interests result mainly from their position in the network, which depends on their relationship with others in this network and on various social and cognitive factors.[29] A major requirement for knowledge to become accepted as a scientific fact involves the option to link this information to practices outside the laboratory that are regarded as a social need.

This study describes the conditions in the network that were conducive to influencing the interactions and the groups that were able to benefit from them: when, why, and how groups or individuals became participants in the network for establishing knowledge of biological masculinity and femininity based on the organization theory. It also describes changes in these conditions, the consequent strengthening or weakening of the different groups or individuals within the network, and the resulting effect on their influence of interactions between 1959 and 1985.

In this analysis from a social network perspective, the images of masculinity and femininity in accepted knowledge represent the historical and social processes involved in the interactions between biomedical scientists, physicians, psychologists, psychiatrists, feminists, and sociologists. The changing conditions affecting the internal dynamics of the distinct groups or individuals in the network have led to continuous reconstruction of the images of masculinity and femininity in interactions or negotiations about acceptance of knowledge concerning development of behavior.

During the period covered by this study, the views among those involved in the network varied considerably regarding the importance of nature for the development of human behavior. This study explores the reconstruction of images of masculinity and femininity as well as of the dividing line between nature and nurture within the network in interactions about the acceptance of knowledge.

Up to this point, I have mentioned biomedical scientists, physicians, psychologists, and psychiatrists who worked with the prenatal hormone paradigm in research or medical practice. Their relation to this knowledge is relatively straightforward. They operate at the core of the network in which knowledge about biological femininity and masculinity is accepted. Surrounding this nucleus are other groups whose relation to this knowledge is more complicated or indirect: feminists of different generations.

Most feminists oppose biological explanations for the differences in behavior between women and men. A minority of feminists, however, did not oppose these explanations. Some feminists participated directly in interactions about the acceptance of knowledge as women researchers studying hormone effects on the development of behavior. Feminist biologists and feminist philosophers criticized the knowledge of biological effects on behavior. Some of these feminist philosophers also inspired me to analyze the contextual history of the development of knowledge in behavioral neuroendocrinology with the insights they had developed. The following introduction of different groups of feminists also includes the theoretical background to questions discussed in the following chapters.

Feminist Visions of Biological Sex Differences

The cultural feminists, as Alice Echols has chosen to call them, argue that women differ from men because their lives are different, and because different experiences result in a different female nature.[30] Cultural feminists often implicitly refer to a biological explanation. For example, motherhood would imply that women are by nature more pacifist than men. Women might also have their own sexuality or way of thinking and learning. The aim of cultural feminists is to revaluate femininity. Their designation of femininity as superior to masculinity contradicts most descriptions of these qualities, including biological reports. For example, they consider a nurturing and emotional nature to be more valuable to humanity than a dominant and rational disposition. Cultural feminists argue that women are actually the stronger sex since they outlive men by an average of six to seven years and because these feminists consider giving birth more heroic than the types of heroism ascribed to males (especially in war situations).[31] Cultural feminism, however, is not homogeneous, and biological explanations of differences given by some of them are not universally accepted among the group. The key link between cultural feminists is their tendency to invoke universalizing conceptions of women and mothers in an essentialist way.[32]

The majority of feminists, however, consider this emphasis on the differences between women and men undesirable. They suggest that championing a redefined "womanhood" would not benefit the development of a useful long-term program for feminism and might even create obstacles. According to most feminists, the highly valued feminine strengths arose from restrictions on freedom. Most of all, they fear biological explanations for sex differences because of the determinism they imply. Based on the classical ideas of genetic determinism, they assume it is impossible to change conditions determined by biology. Only social conditions are receptive to change.

The political demands of most feminists extend beyond a reassessment of "female values"; they opt for radical social change. These feminists' aversion to biologism is strengthened by the unflattering biological statements about women's intellectual capacities that had impeded their access to universities in the past.[33] Although they are from different eras and varying levels of radicalism, most feminists designate those counterparts who believe in a different female nature as "essentialists," which most feminists consider a derogatory term. Cultural feminists and other feminists agree, however, on the need for change in women's social positions and lives. Their main difference is over the support among cultural feminists for postulating biological sex differences, which the majority of feminists oppose.

In the footsteps of Beauvoir and others, mainstream feminists have developed social and psychoanalytical theories to investigate and to change the oppression of women, the asymmetrical positions of women and men in society, and many other feminist subjects mentioned during the second feminist wave.

Feminist Ideology Haunted by Biology

Feminists' aversions to biological ideas concerning the concepts of female and male have influenced their positions in the network of biomedical scientists investigating the development of femininity and masculinity in behavior and the theoretical views developed about this subject. Based on the work of Simone de Beauvoir and Margaret Mead, the majority of feminists have considered biology unimportant for understanding the development of femininity and masculinity in the behavior and social positions of women and men. Strategic considerations have led feminists to exclude biological notions from their theories. Feminist scholars view the difference between biological *sex* and cultural or psychosocial *gender* as the most important distinction. The words "female," a "woman," and "male," a "man," refer to unchangeable and universal sex and biology: These terms have been excluded from feminist theory. Femininity and masculinity refer to gender and are considered sociocultural constructs and thus subject to change.[34] Feminist theory and research deal with gender, which includes sexuality, and questions the mechanisms that construct the link between sex and gender.

The insight that "woman" and "femininity" do not necessarily occur together led feminist scholars to question the dual concepts of masculinity and femininity[35] and to propose several alternative role models that are *androgynous* (a term that combines the Greek words *andros* and *gunaikos,* meaning man and woman, respectively). These models allow men and women to develop characteristics traditionally associated with the other sex. The androgynous models elicited a debate within feminism in which feminists who found it more important to stress the differences and to revaluate femininity argued that androgyny was normative for women. Androgyny would fit women into a cultural ideal that conflicted with the feminine, as its ideal implied the adoption of masculinity by women. Moreover, they argued, these models implicitly accepted that characteristics associated with femininity were socially inferior. Advocates of the androgyny models argued against the existence of "the feminine," which they viewed as the result of oppression. They chose androgyny (although it was considered an individual trait, rather than a social structure) for strategic reasons: to avoid biological determinism or essentialism.

This description is a very general recapitulation of the discussion.[36] There has been considerable debate about the political implications of choices between models that emphasize difference between genders and models that emphasize plurality within gender.[37]

In feminist theory, the relationship between differences and determinism remains problematic. On the one hand, a frequent criticism holds that feminist theory presupposes a biological basis for the phenomena that have been explained. Many debates in feminism deal with precultural, essentialist, or biological differences.[38] On the other hand, feminists' negation of any explanation involving determination by biology leads to the view that masculinity and femininity result entirely from cultural factors. The very existence of intentions not determined by cultural circumstances is questioned. Some feminist theories are reproached for replacing a biological explanation for social phenomena, thus leading from biologism to culturalism or nominalism.[39]

Notwithstanding these debates and outbursts of criticism, feminist theory and research have been tremendously successful in producing knowledge about the social and psychological mechanisms involved in the oppression of women or social inequality between women and men. Until the late 1970s, however, feminist theory shunned biology.

The issue of hormones and oral contraceptives reflected the feminist dilemma surrounding biology. On the one hand, the scientific explanation of women's reproductive functions in terms of hormonal functions had a side effect that was of particular interest to women and especially to feminists. Oral contraceptives meant that women could enjoy sex without fear of pregnancy and could decide for the first time in history whether or not to become mothers. Many women found that hormones taken at the right time in the correct doses prevented pregnancy. This discovery established faith in knowledge about hormones. Aside from oral contraceptives, women took hormones for all other problems scientifically connected to the reproductive system, such as premenstrual, menstrual, and menopausal disorders. In the 1970s, however, studies increasingly questioned the effectiveness of some of these hormone treatments. Premenstrual disorders and menopausal problems were attributed to psychological causes that could not be solved by hormones. Moreover, some of these hormone treatments were associated with an increased risk of cancer. Feminists expressed contradictory views of hormone treatments. In England, they demanded that physicians take female health issues seriously and asked for estrogen replacement therapy for menopausal complaints. Feminists in the United States argued that hormone therapy would lead to medicalization and stereotyping of women according to their biology.[40] Although the arguments were contradictory, medical intervention based on knowledge about hormonal regulation of women's reproductive systems affected the bodies and lives of practically all women in Western societies.

Ambivalent opinions about hormone treatments and stereotypes regarding the hormonal impact on differences in behavior were especially difficult for feminists to accept. As a consequence, some feminists stopped ignoring biology and became involved in interactions concerning the acceptance of knowledge about hormone effects.

Biological Ideology Haunted by Feminism

Feminists' involvement in the acceptance of knowledge concerning hormones varied. I have distinguished three groups according to their views concerning the allegation that biomedical investigations provide truth about human nature.

The first group agreed that experimental research helped reveal the true causes of differences in behavioral development between women and men. In the early 1970s, women began to enter science in increasing numbers.[41] They were educated within the biomedical disciplines and adopted the assumptions of the subdisciplines in which they were educated.[42] Before the 1970s, women scientists were exceptions and were rarely in a position to generate theories, to ask research questions, or to develop research designs. While some women did produce original insights, their ideas were mostly credited to their male supervisors or colleagues.[43] Since they became common actors in scientific practice in the 1970s, women have contributed to scientific development in the field of behavioral neuroendocrinology and other disciplines involved in the question of sex differences.

Since the late 1970s, another group of feminists, educated within the biological disciplines, has challenged the "truth" of scientific knowledge and has argued that one-sided views and gender bias in issues concerning research and methods of investigation provided a scientific truth that did not accord with women's experiences. During this period, ideology in science has become a popular subject. Its sources include publications by sociologists and philosophers from the Frankfurt School and the work of Michel Foucault.[44] Feminist scholars adopted these ideas and published analyses of biological investigations from the perspective that science, the general production of knowledge, is a political activity. In *Biological Politics,* psychologist Janet Sayers submits that recent research on prenatal hormone effects on human brain development and behavior parallel nineteenth-century research on differences in brain size in the production of arguments that bar women from effective social participation. During the first feminist wave, women's demands for suffrage and access to universities were rejected on the basis of arguments from craniometrics: The average size of a woman's brain was smaller than a man's brain, and women's smaller brains could not provide them with sufficient intelligence to vote or to study.[45] Feminist biologists, including Ruth Hubbard, Ruth Bleier, Anne Fausto-Sterling, and Lynda Birke, argue that biological investigations into sex differences have produced knowledge that contributes to maintaining the status quo. In biological investigations, women (and non-Caucasians) appear to be biologically inferior or passive, which makes their social subordination seem natural.[46]

I will return to the criticism of feminist biologists that is relevant to my analysis of the development of research based on the organization theory. First, these feminist biologists provided a *methodological* critique of the production of knowledge about the biological background of female nature and behavior that was based on one-sided biological research. This methodological critique considered the questions scientists selected for their research as well as their approach to investigating these questions. The philosopher Helen Longino described a method for examining the methodology of biological research for signs of gender bias.[47] She and the feminists mentioned above scrutinized several fields in biology, such as evolutionary biology, neurology, and endocrinology, for their ideological presuppositions about women and men in research. Their main point of criticism originated from the feminist theory that only social environment can explain sex differences in behavior and that biological factors are irrelevant. These feminists also argued that the neglect or underestimation of environmental factors in interpreting the results distorted the importance of the effects ascribed to biological factors (e.g., prenatal hormones in research based on the organization theory).

Feminist biologists admitted that hormones could affect behavior, but they considered biological differences less important than biologists did. Nobody believed that current research methods could distinguish between hormonal and environmental effects, or that they could establish the effects of prenatal and other hormones on human behavior.

Lynda Birke used this argument to describe the possibility for developing a new research model in which biological and environmental factors and behavior affect one another. All variables in this model interact and result in a dynamic concept of gender (behavior). According to this model, behavior is not necessarily the outcome of biology or the environment. Rather, behavior can affect these spheres.

Second, feminist biologists criticized the *extrapolation* of the results from experiments with hormones from laboratory animals to human behavior. Bleier argued that the effects of prenatal hormones on the behavior of related laboratory animals (e.g., rats and hamsters) differed considerably. Questions arose regarding the validity of any animal model for investigating prenatal hormone effects in humans.

Third, Bleier criticized the limitations attributed by scientists to the effects of hormones. She believed all sorts of hormones are present during fetal development in most animals and humans and that this makes it difficult to ascertain the precise effect of a specific type of hormone on a certain species or sex. For the same reason, she suggested that extrapolations from one species to the other about the effects of prenatal hormones on behavior are incorrect, certainly for the biological understanding of human behavior. This criticism revealed the importance of methodology as a vehicle for the phenomenon of androcentric bias or ideology. It also suggested that biological research based on another methodology could be free of gender bias (ideology) and that a single truth about biological sex differences is knowable.

How did the criticism of feminist biologists affect their general position in the interactions with biomedical investigators about the acceptance of knowledge? To many biomedical scientists, feminist biologists seemed to adopt a "male conspiracy" perspective in their criticism of biological research on sex differences. Understandably, this impression did not improve the relationship between feminists and biomedical scientists. Most of the critical arguments included a remark such as that made by Anne Fausto-Sterling:

> Scientists in analyzing male/female differences peer through the prism of everyday culture. More often than not their hidden agendas that are unarticulated, bear strong resemblances to broader social agendas. Although no one can be entirely successful, all serious scientists strive to eliminate such blind spots. The prospects of success diminish enormously, however, when the area of research touches one very personally. And what could be more personally significant than our sense of ourselves as female or male? In the study of gender it is impossible for any individual to do unbiased research.[48]

In this passage, Fausto-Sterling comes across as rather charitable toward all scientists involved in gender research (femininity and masculinity in behavior), although the "hidden agendas" can be assumed to refer to subconscious or even conscious meanings.

Aside from their difficulties with the "conspiracy" perspectives, scientists were irritated by the arguments of feminist biologists criticizing science for male bias. In the first place, they implied that this research was not as objective as scientists had led the public to believe. Biological research, however, derives part of its status from its reputation for objectivity. In general, biomedical scientists complied with this demand for the standards considered necessary for respectable scientific practice. In the second place, this gender-biased lack of objectivity was socially incorrect in the circles of progressive scientists with the best intentions for progress in understanding human nature and other forms of nature, particularly in the 1970s and 1980s.

To give the reader an idea of the interaction between feminist critics of biology and biologists, I would like to provide some examples. If you ask any feminist biologist you will find that there are many more examples. In 1984 the scientists Dick Swaab and Michel Hofman from the Dutch Brain Institute published an article reacting to feminist criticism; they explicitly opposed the feminist author Germaine Greer. In 1970 she provided strong arguments against biologism, the tendency to explain sex differences in behavior by biological differences, in her book *The Female Eunuch*.[49] Swaab and Hofman gave an overview of all sorts of sex differences in the human brain. These included microscopic structures in the brain but also brain weight and size, which are, on average, smaller in women. In their discussion Swaab and Hofman regressed to nineteenth-century thought in connecting the amount of brain tissue with intelligence, thus suggesting that women are less intelligent than men.[50]

A third group of feminists can be identified for their vision of scientific truth. According to feminist philosophers of science such as Evelyn Fox Keller, Sandra Harding, and many others who deal with epistemological questions about scientific inquiry, gendered science is not merely a question of methodology. They question whether science is an inherently masculine project. Harding argues that "masculine" scientists have historically been concerned with distinguishing themselves from members of the other sex. She submits that this concern underlies the preoccupation among male investigators with finding the continuities between men and males from other species and between women and females from other species.[51] Accordingly, Keller argues that the scientific demand for objectivity is a product of masculine psychological development.[52] These feminist philosophers thus suspect that gendered science involves deeper layers in science than in methodology. For example, Keller explains that acceptance of scientific theories is influenced by the sex of the investigators who develop them. Using examples from physics and genetics, she also argues that theories in accordance with dominant images of masculinity tend to be accepted more easily by the scientific community than theories that defy or diverge from such images.[53] The next chapter will examine whether and in what manner the acceptance of the organization theory was ruled by this principle.

Feminist biologist Ruth Bleier's opinion differs slightly from the views of feminist philosophers Keller and Harding. Bleier claims that our perception of truth is affected by the cultural division into femininity and masculinity. She formulates the problem as follows: "The historical separation of human experience into mutually contradictory realms, female and male, engendered our culturally inherited dualistic mode of thought, and that male-female dichotomy was built into our ways of perceiving truth."[54]

Helen Longino does not consider feminists immune to this way of thinking. She even believes they helped perpetuate the dualistic mode of thinking about femininity and masculinity:

> As long as feminists counter theories of biological determination of gender difference and sexual orientation with competing environmental explanations of their origin, the discussion will revolve around the dimorphic center. As long as it does so, biologically oriented scientists and thinkers will continue to advance biological determinist theories. As long as they do, dimorphism will remain unexamined as reality and as ideal. As long as dimorphism remains an ideal, individuals will attempt to conform to it. And, finally, as long as individuals attempt to conform to it, dimorphism will appear to be enough of a reality to require explanation. As long as dimorphism remains at the center of discourse, other patterns of difference remain hidden both as possibility and as reality.[55]

Ruth Bleier considers it important for feminists to question and examine all dualisms, all dichotomous ways in which nature, human "nature," and human activities are described, analyzed, and categorized. She also feels that universal concepts and modes of thinking have damaged science and scholarship in other areas by structuring our social world and the role of women in this world. Evidently, research based on the organization theory provides knowledge that subjects human nature to a dualist categorization: Biomedical researchers speak of "sex dimorphism" in behavior.[56]

The main theme of this study should therefore be reformulated as follows: How did scientists and physicians construct *dualistic* images of femininity and masculinity by producing knowledge based on the organization theory? How did feminism help stabilize or change these images? The answers to these questions use a social network approach to consider the development of knowledge on the basis of the proposal of the organization theory about differentiation of the brain.

Toward Constructing Masculinity and Femininity in a Network

A constructivist perspective would view science as a social activity and knowledge as a social product and would attribute the meaning of both science and knowledge to a certain period and place. Sociologists of science who subscribe to constructivism therefore suggest that scientific knowledge is the product of social, political, and economic negotiations, rather than of empirical discovery: Scientists are not discovering reality, they are actively constructing reality.[57]

In the 1980s, feminists investigating the history of science from this perspective, such as Londa Schiebinger and Ludmilla Jordanova, explored the cultural intertwinement of science with sex and sexuality. Schiebinger described reflections of parts of the body that were politically significant in nineteenth-century anatomical drawings. In drawings of female skeletons, the pelvis is very wide, whereas the skull is relatively small, thereby conveying the importance these anatomists attached to those parts of women's bodies for child bearing and intellectual activities, respectively.[58] Jordanova analyzed in detail professional and popular medical and biological writings, sculptures, anatomical wax models, paintings, films, poetry, and fiction to demonstrate how scientific ideas can be understood as "mediations," containing implications beyond their explicit content. She described the central role of fluid and ever-changing opposites, such as male versus female and reason versus emotion, in the culture of science as well as their power as images in their own right.[59]

Donna Haraway and Susan Bell explored the intertwinement of political and social interests with biological and medical concepts of masculinity and femininity embodied in recent scientific concepts and theories. Haraway analyzed knowledge produced in primatology (ethological studies of monkeys),[60] and Bell focused on hormone treatments for women.[61] These studies highlighted the impact of macrosociological and power relations concerning women and men on the acceptance of scientific results and practices.

Anthropologists and sociologists of science, such as Latour and Woolgar, focused on local conditions in sites where knowledge was produced (laboratories and medical practices) and on the effects of accidental conditions on processes that reconstructed the significance of the subjects under investigation.[62] These studies developed the social network approach.

Nelly Oudshoorn used a social network approach to analyze the contextual history of the development of sex endocrinology in the 1920s and 1930s.[63] She unraveled the interactions between laboratory scientists, gynecologists, and pharmaceutical entrepreneurs involved in producing knowledge about female and male sex hormones and their pharmaceutical production. Her study described the cultural notions of masculinity and femininity that guided the different groups in developing scientific facts and the changes that these ideas underwent after their incorporation into scientific and clinical tests. The actions of laboratory scientists, gynecologists, and pharmaceutical entrepreneurs reconstructed the meanings of sex differences from anatomical (ovaries or testes) to chemical (female or male hormones) in nature. Oudshoorn elegantly demonstrated the dependence of these groups on material conditions and existing organizational structures in the 1920s and 1930s. The availability of resources for research on "female" hormones increased the focus on such investigations. Whereas "female" hormones from the urine of females were easily obtainable as a consequence of existing gynecological practice, the male equivalent of andrology developed only in the 1970s. Gynecological practices also served as markets for pharmaceutical hormone products. Thus, different groups focusing on female hormones and applications of hormone treatments for a broad range of female diseases sustained and perpetuated ideas and practices in Western culture that were responsible for subjecting female bodies to medical interventions more easily than male bodies. Oudshoorn's study described the conditions that benefited these laboratory scientists, gynecologists, and pharmaceutical entrepreneurs and their role in changing images of masculinity and femininity once they became embedded in science and science-based practices. Her study covers an era in which cultural ideas of femininity and masculinity went unquestioned.

The present study deals with a period in which femininity and masculinity are questioned and the effect of these questions on the conditions and interactions in a network in which knowledge of the development of masculinity and femininity in behavior gained acceptance.

Possibilities and Constraints

What insight can be derived from a network analysis based on a constructivist perspective of science, and what must remain unmentioned? Since Thomas Kuhn's *Structure of Scientific Revolutions* was published in 1962, the tendency of social factors to affect the development of science has gained credence.[64] Recent sociological analysis of scientific development has abandoned the distinction between social processes and cognitive developments in science. The constructivist perspective views science as a social process. This principle means that development of knowledge (the scientific content) is structured by the social context in which this process occurs. Simultaneously, this knowledge is embodied in the social context. According to this perspective, the development of knowledge in a certain period can be the object of science-sociological analysis. Although most scientists accept that research concepts and results have changed in every scientific field over the past thirty years, not all those changes will appeal to the imagination as strongly as ideas and concepts of femininity and masculinity. These changes enable us to consider the development of research based on the organization theory as a normal occurrence in science. Analyzing a scientific development as a normal evolution within a particular social context means that this analysis cannot distinguish between "wrong" or "right" science, or "false" or "true" conclusions. Although such a distinction might be made from a modern—and possibly from a feminist—perspective, it could also be considered an example of Whig history.

Over the past thirty years, beliefs about femininity and masculinity have evolved rapidly. Accordingly, scientific findings concerning femininity and masculinity in behavior that were considered established or true in the 1960s have been abandoned in the 1990s. In the course of three decades, both constructivists and biomedical scientists have become unable to speak about truth without mentioning when the idea in question was valid (when it was meaningful or scientifically accepted and by whom). In the analysis from a constructivist perspective, truth as such does not exist. Moreover, truth is not discovered but is made or constructed by science. This point of view can be difficult for those adhering to convergent realism: Progress resulting from the internal dynamics of science can lead to new discoveries and better knowledge. Constructivism regards science as a project, as it does knowledge, as social phenomena. Therefore, science's internal dynamics are also regarded as science-sociological processes.

The argument in this book is not based on gender bias, which belongs to a positivist perspective, which views science as producing objective truth. The constructivist perspective on science assigns a meaning to scientific truth within a certain time and place. While scientific truth plays a role in that particular context, it is not necessarily significant in another context. When the cultural context changes quickly, scientific truth usually has a rapid turnover as well. This principle applies to biological femininity and masculinity and to a wide range of other issues, such as environmental problems.

This study describes the events that transpired in biomedical knowledge about the development of femininity and masculinity in brains and behavior. It reveals the reacting agents and the parties that expressed criticism, as well as the targets of these acts, the results of the discussions and interactions, and ways to interpret the mechanisms involved in these interactions.

Choosing an actor network perspective on the development of a scientific field generally provides insight into the mechanisms and conditions underlying acceptance of knowledge among the different groups involved. Examining the mechanisms and conditions involved in acceptance of knowledge and reconstructing images of femininity and masculinity may offer perspectives on active and strategic participation in the acceptance of knowledge and the reconstruction of images of femininity and masculinity.

Why the Brain?

The organization theory concerning brain differentiation was expounded from 1959 until approximately 1985; its impact on the course of research serves as a case study for answering the questions outlined in this chapter. The focus of the book is twofold: It attempts to address behavioral neuroendocrinology both as a scientific idea system whose development can be traced through scientific publications that appeared during this period and in terms of the professional contributions and the conditions under which individual scientists produced those publications. This body of knowledge brings together sex and gender, nature and nurture, male and female, and masculinity and femininity in behavior and therefore offers promise for theorizing about sex and gender. The political interest of this case on macro- and microlevels is even more important. Throughout history, differences in the brain have played a role in political issues, although the rhetoric has become more subtle since the turn of the twentieth century, when differences in the volume of male and female skulls were seen as a parameter for differences in intelligence. The Italian anthropologist and historian Gianna Pomata has suggested that the boundaries of the sex roles in our culture are sustained by biological investigations into sex differences. Other cultures enforce absolute separation of the sexes through rituals in which only men or women participate. In Western culture, the confines of sex roles are less rigid, and competition between individuals of different sexes is theoretically possible. Pomata argues that biomedical explanations concerning sex differences serve the same purpose as rituals among tribes in New Guinea to maintain separate domains for men and women.[65] In our society, competition affects people with new and unorthodox ambitions, such as women seeking careers in science and technology and men interested in caring for their children. Popular writing about differential capacities of women and men due to sex differences in the brain suggest that such wishes are not in accord with a female or male nature. In many cases these articles confirm traditional stereotypes of women and men. They color people's views of themselves and others, mostly in a negative sense. One of my students provided an example of this outlook. She was complaining about her lack of progress in her studies and suggested that the problem might involve her female brain, as it was less capable of abstract thought than the minds of her male friends studying biology. Was she verbalizing a more general thought? Would she have chosen this explanation if she had never heard or read about sex differences in the brain and their consequences for the abilities of males and females? I doubt it.

This study deals with knowledge concerning the boundaries of biological sex and cultural gender. Gender and sex are present on the levels that Keller distinguished in *Reflections on Gender and Science*. On the first level, gender and sex serve as a metaphor, as an ideology in science signifying the development and acceptance of the theory about differentiation of the brain. The second level involves the construction of male and female brains and masculinity and femininity in behavior by scientists, doctors, and psychiatrists for producing and using knowledge about behavioral neuroendocrinology. The third level addresses the identities of male and female scientists. In this study, mixing terms belonging to discourse either about sex or about gender is unavoidable. I will use the words male and female for biological topics and the words masculinity and femininity subjects related to gender. Descriptions that deviate from this rule will inevitably appear. The following chapters will unravel the methods of interaction between sex and gender on these three levels.

As the chapters in this book have been designed as independent units, the overlap between the information on the research on animals based on the organization theory and its implications for humans is limited. Chapter 2 focuses on the period 1959–1972: the acceptance of the theory by biomedical scientists and its extension from animal behavior to human behavior. It reveals the development of knowledge based on the theory and the conditions that led scientists in the field to accept this knowledge.

Chapter 3 focuses on research developments of the 1970s and 1980s and the influence of feminism on this process. It reconstructs the conditions of the events that stabilized or changed the concepts scientists used in their experiments for investigating prenatal hormone effects on the development of masculinity and femininity in behavior.

Chapter 4 relates the applications of the knowledge described in chapters 2 and 3 by physicians and psychiatrists in treating people born as intersex to help them become "real" women or men (both anatomically and psychologically) and the possibilities for and constraints against changing this treatment.

Finally, chapter 5 evaluates the lessons of this study regarding the construction of masculinity and femininity in behavioral neuroendocrinology. Moreover, I will fulfill some theoretical promises made in this introductory chapter.

2

ACCEPTANCE OF SCIENTIFIC THEORIES AND IMAGES OF MASCULINITY AND FEMININITY

Introduction

In 1972 scientists completed their biological explanation for differences in male and female behavior. In the period between 1959 and 1972 they reconstructed ideas about masculinity and femininity by considering the way people behave as a result of prenatal hormones acting on the developing brain. Scientists based their experiments on the *organization theory* proposed in 1959. According to this theory, the development of a male brain and masculine behavior requires androgens prior to birth, whereas the development of a female brain and feminine behavior does not.[1]

We will see how the acceptance of the organization theory resulted from the theory's reliance on culturally prevalent images of masculinity and femininity.[2] These images turn out to be associated with the functions of "male" and "female" hormones. First we will examine the events that followed its introduction.

Introduction and Context of the Proposal of the Organization Theory

In 1959, Charles Phoenix, Robert Goy, Arnold Gerall, and William Young postulated the organization hypothesis of brain differentiation. They all worked for the Department of Anatomy at the University of Kansas. Young was a professor in the department; Phoenix, Goy, and Gerall were postgraduate fellows. During the 1950s, Young had worked in embryology as well as with psychologists, and his scientific ideas reflected his contacts with both fields.[3] The organization theory can therefore be regarded as an integrative theory, since it brings together ideas from two different fields.[4]

The organization hypothesis carefully distinguishes the early "organizational" effects of hormones on brain tissue (either immediately before birth or in the first few days thereafter, depending on the species) from their "activational" effects (the effects of these hormones on fully developed neural mechanisms in adult animals).[5] Before the advent of the organization hypothesis, scientists had believed that gonadal hormones exerted temporary effects on sexual behavior in adult organisms. The introduction of the organization theory enabled research to be conducted on the permanent effects of hormones on early brain development (expressed in behavioral characteristics). Based on their experiments with hormones administered to guinea pigs before birth, the Kansas investigators posited the following hypothesis: "Androgenic substances received prenatally have an organizing action on the tissues mediating mating behavior in the sense of altering permanently the responses females normally give as adults, resulting in masculine mating behavior."[6]

This hypothesis provided the first clear theoretical framework for the experimental results of the effects of prenatal hormones on behavior.[7] Its formulation made it possible to measure brain differentiation by observing sexual behavior. According to the theory, male behavior develops only when androgens are present before birth. Male behavior was defined by this hypothesis in terms of "mounting": one animal climbing onto another animal's back. When there are no androgens, female sexual behavior develops. Female behavior was defined as arching of the back; the scientists called this behavior "lordosis" and regarded it as a sign of receptivity. In natural situations, both types of behavior occur among both sexes of most animals: males and females can be tested on displays of mounting as well as on displays of lordosis.

To convey the context in which the organization theory was proposed, I will rely on the article published by its originators in 1959. Phoenix, Goy, Gerall, and Young referred to research from the 1930s and 1940s. The first investigations into the prenatal effects of hormones had occurred during the 1930s, and experiments concerning the effects of hormones on mating behavior had been reported by Carroll A. Pfeiffer (1936) at the Zoological Laboratory of the University of Iowa and by Vera Dantchakoff and Albert Raynaud (1938) in France. These scientists castrated different rodents at birth and/or injected them with different types of hormones and studied their later sexual behavior. They had suggested that androgens (regarded as male hormones) and estrogens (regarded as female hormones) had identical effects on mating behavior of rats.[8] Studies in the 1930s hypothesized a kind of sensitization for later hormones. Phoenix and his colleagues, however, believed that "unexplored since (these) studies . . . is the possibility that androgens or estrogens reaching animals' brains during the prenatal period might have an *organizing* action that would be reflected by the character of adult sexual behavior."[9] Here, organizing means that the effects are structural and permanent.

During the late 1930s, scientists had argued that both types of hormones that reached the brains of animals during the perinatal period might affect the central nervous system. The studies conducted in the 1930s are, in fact, remarkably similar to those performed after 1959. There are, however, a few essential differences. While in the 1930s *both* androgens and estrogens were thought to influence brain differentiation and behavior, the hormones held responsible for this process had been narrowed down to testosterone (or some metabolite of testosterone) twenty years later. In 1959, a theory was proposed about *permanent* prenatal hormonal effects on brain differentiation, a possibility that had long been rejected. What led to this proposal?

The proposal of the organization theory can be attributed in part to developments in another discipline. In the 1940s, embryologists studied hormonal effects on embryonic differentiation of the genital tract. In the early 1950s, experimental research performed by Alfred Jost, who had worked at the Collège de France in Paris since the 1940s, suggested that organisms developed male genitals when androgens were present and female genitals when androgens were absent.[10]

In the same period, researchers also tried to understand the hormonal mechanisms underlying the function of the ovarian cycle. They found that regulation of the ovaries in rats (by hormones from the pituitary gland) was mediated by the brain, specifically, by the hypothalamus. Furthermore, this part of the brain produced so-called releasing factors in a cyclical way in females and in a constant or tonic way in males. The next logical step involved questioning how the hypothalamus of the female rodent differed from that of the male. It appeared that when males were deprived of androgens through castration at birth, their pattern of producing releasing factors could be made cyclical by administering estrogens in later life, provided that the testes were removed within five to seven days after birth. Based on these results, researchers concluded that androgens had an "organizing" effect on fetal rat brains during this period, and that characteristically "female" brains developed in the absence of circulating androgens.[11]

These investigations in embryology led scientists to believe that the female condition is the basic state and that the development of the male sexual apparatus and a constant production of releasing factors by the hypothalamus is caused by androgens and represents a modification of this primary condition. Before these investigations, embryonal organisms had been considered bisexual. Some researchers now call the effects of androgens on males the "Adam Principle," meaning that "to differentiate a male something must be added."[12]

The organization hypothesis was explicitly proposed in analogy to the results of Jost's experiments on the embryonic differentiation of the genital tract. Researchers thought that the development of the male brain was organized by androgens and that the female brain, since it was not organized by androgens, was "basic." Neuroendocrinologists adopted the Adam Principle in preference to the idea from the 1930s that androgens and estrogens both affected brain differentiation.

Acceptance and Extension of the Organization Theory

After 1959, many scientists started mentioning the organizational aspects of brain differentiation in their articles. Phoenix and his colleagues had performed their experiments on guinea pigs. In the early 1960s, much research was published on the validity of their hypothesis with regard to other rodents; investigations of mating behavior in rats and other laboratory animals (e.g., mice and hamsters) were performed after hormonal manipulations, such as castration at birth or administration of sex hormones.[13] By 1964, the organization hypothesis had evolved into a theory about the origin of sexual behavior, and many articles referred to it as "a concept."[14] The theory was subsequently extended to other types of behavior and would soon be applied to human behavior as well.

In 1964, three of the authors of the original article published a paper on the theory's validity with regard to rhesus monkeys, the animal species considered most closely related to humans.[15] By this time, Phoenix and his colleagues, Young and Goy, worked in the Reproductive Physiology and Behavior section of the Oregon Regional Primate Research Center in Beaverton, Oregon. They had already announced the importance of the theory for understanding human behavior in their initial proposal. Later, Goy stated that switching experimental animals from rodents to monkeys reflected the interest of scientists in relating the theoretical implications of the organization theory to human behavior.[16]

The 1964 article explained behavioral differences between male and female monkeys in terms of the organization theory. The authors argued again that the theory was important for explaining human sexuality: "In

our opinion the many differences in behavior which in the growing child
and adult are socially rather than hormonally determined have obscured
the possible role of the hormones in maintaining the strength of the sexual
drive."[17] Though the experiments tested the behavior of only two monkeys, the article initiated a new line of investigation.

Since 1965, scientists from several disciplines, including psychology,
have published research on the prenatal effects of hormones on all kinds
of sex-dimorphic behavior in various animals, including human beings.[18]
The following list gives the reader an impression of the varieties of
noncoital behaviors supposedly affected by prenatal hormone exposure:[19]

in rodents
maternal nest-building[20]
running wheel activity
open field activity
shock elicited aggression
isolation induced aggression
taste preferences
feeding and body weight
active avoidance learning
maze learning[21]

in birds
nest-building
song learning

in monkeys
rough and tumble play
dominance

In fact, less than ten years after its introduction, the organization
theory was used in investigations of human behavior. In the United States,
psychologists John Money and Anke Ehrhardt extended the theory to
include human behavior. Money was a professor of medical psychology
and pediatrics at Johns Hopkins Hospital in Baltimore, and Ehrhardt was
an associate professor of psychiatry with the Division of Child Psychiatry
at the College of Physicians and Surgeons of Columbia University. Since
the 1950s, these scientists had been working with children born with
ambiguous genitals, a phenomenon that could be explained within Jost's

theory of the effect of hormones on genital development. Jost's experiments provided an understanding of genital intersexuality in both animals and humans and resolved an issue that had been a subject of research since the beginning of the twentieth century: Children born as intersex individuals, previously regarded as a punishment or a sign from God, or as an impossible third sex, became a transparent and manipulable manifestation of a disturbed regulation of hormones.

Money and Ehrhardt advocated surgical correction of the genitals as soon as possible after birth to ensure normal psychological development. Initially, they believed that psychosexual development occurred after birth. After the appearance of the theory on sexual differentiation of the brain (which was analogous to the theory of genital development), they considered people born with ambiguous genitals to be experiments of nature in the sense that their existence made it possible to investigate whether their brains had also been affected by the prenatal hormonal disturbance. Their psychosexual development was examined in the light of the organization theory.

In 1972, Money and Ehrhardt published a book on the results of their studies on sexual and other behavior of children born as intersex.[22] Best known are their findings regarding CAH girls, or "tomboys"—girls born with masculinized genitalia due to the production of abnormal hormones by the adrenal gland before birth. The usual medical practice involved surgical correction of the genitalia of these girls to female.[23] Money and Ehrhardt found that these girls were more active than the children of the control group: they liked to play with boys, had a "high energy expenditure," enjoyed "rough and tumble play," preferred practical clothing to pretty dresses, and had fantasies about a career instead of motherhood. Other findings included a tendency toward the development of a higher IQ, as well as a tendency toward a bisexual or lesbian sexual orientation, the result of masculinization of their brains by androgens. Money and Ehrhardt argued that although social environment is important, biological factors before birth should not be ignored.

These investigations *reproduced* the social image of masculinity (and males) and associated masculinity with active behavior, career, and intelligence, whereas femininity (and female behavior) was associated with passivity, motherhood, and a lower intelligence level than males. At the same time, the investigations based on the organization theory *produced* or *constructed* an image of a biological background that formed the basis for masculinity and femininity and was attributed to the result of hormonal action on the fetal brain. Homosexuality was also connected to the organization theory, and it was claimed that this phenomenon could also be understood as the effect of a hormonal disturbance before birth. Günther Dörner, the director of the Institute of Experimental Endocrinology at Humboldt University in Berlin (German Democratic Republic), suggested hormone treatments for women considered at risk for giving birth to a homosexual son.[24]

Despite the acceptance and extension of the organization theory to fields beyond sexual behavior, as well as to humans, opposition arose. The primary critic was Frank Beach, chair of the Psychology Department of the University of California at Berkeley. Beach had been investigating hormone effects on behavior since the 1940s and had always been highly influential in this field.[25] In 1971, he published an ironic and critical article in which he argued that methodological problems and issues concerning conflicting results of experiments based on the organization theory remained unresolved.[26] Beach was among the few scientists who did not subscribe to the organization theory. At least, he was the scholar who published his objections. Notwithstanding Beach's severe criticism, in 1972 Money and Ehrhardt's work established the notion that sex differences in the brain and thus in behavior were caused by gonadal hormones, both in animals and in humans.

The research of Money and Ehrhardt, and especially Dörner's homosexuality prevention treatments, have been criticized by researchers in neuroendocrinology and other fields.[27] In the next section we will see how the idea that homosexuality is due to disturbed prenatal hormones contributed to the acceptance of the organization theory.

Reasons for Acceptance of the Organization Theory

The organization theory marked the beginning of a new period in behavioral endocrinology.[28] The theory's success was remarkable, especially since even the authors acknowledged that the "hypothesis that . . . hormones have an organizing action in the sense of patterning the responses an individual gives to such substances has long been rejected."[29] Why was the organization theory almost universally accepted in 1959?

The reasons for the acceptance of the theory emanate from different aspects of the production of knowledge. Several are of a scientific and philosophical nature, such as the added value the theory gave to knowledge claims, the unification of domains that followed the proposal of the theory, and the fact that the theory correlated with previously accepted knowledge in these fields. The theory's acceptance and, stronger still, its extension to include human behavior can also be viewed according to the social context of the late 1960s and 1970s. At that time the women's movement made an issue of prevailing notions of masculinity and femininity. Another significant factor involved was the different disciplinary status of psychology from biology. While these factors should be noted, they should not be separated, as their interaction furthered the acceptance and production of knowledge based on the organization theory.

First, the proposal of the theory gave scientists a theoretical basis for reinforcing their research claims. In several disciplines, such as embryology and endocrinology, experiments on the effects of hormones and behavior were performed without any theoretical background, since this type of research was still in a formative stage.[30]

Second, the theory connected disciplines that had previously existed as separate entities by giving them a common subject of research. The theory's proposal coincided with the proclamation of its importance to other disciplines. The articles of the 1930s had not had this effect. In 1959, Phoenix and his colleagues addressed both neurology and psychology (i.e., the field of human behavior):

"Neurologists or psychologists interested in the effects of the androgens on neural tissues would hardly think of alterations so drastic. Instead, a more subtle change reflected in function rather than in visible structure would be presumed."[31] Moreover, they argued, "involved in this suggestion is the view that behavior may be treated as a dependent variable and therefore that we may speak of shaping the behavior by hormone administration just as the psychologist speaks of shaping behavior by manipulating the external environment."[32]

This argument has clearly been quite convincing. It has inspired psychiatrists and psychologists, in addition to neurologists, endocrinologists, and scientists from other disciplines with biomedical orientations. Reports of experiments based on the organization theory have appeared in journals with different disciplinary backgrounds.[33] The theory provided a new subject of investigation to these expanding fields of research: the development of masculinity and femininity in the brain. The relevance of research claims based on the organization theory extended beyond the fields in which the experiments had actually been performed. In a period when masculinity and femininity were no longer entities that could be taken for granted, this elasticity was very appealing to researchers. The relevance of prenatal hormones for brain development and later human behavior was explained in textbooks for all biomedical studies, including psychology. Results of investigations concerning masculinity, femininity,

or sex differences in behavior were no longer convincing without referring to the organization theory. In the next chapter we will see how even
feminists subscribed to it. We may say that the organization theory
became "an obligatory point of passage" for anyone involved in investigations of masculinity and femininity in behavior.[34]

John Money and Anke Ehrhardt became important collaborators in
establishing the theory as an "obligatory point of passage." When their
book was published in 1972, the controversy over the impact of genetic
heredity or social environment on the development of male and female
behavior was topical. Genetic research, however, was unable to provide
specific answers to questions about the origin of behavioral patterns. It
proved impossible to develop an experimental design for both animals
and humans in which genetic material could be controlled and the
behavioral outcome tested. The organization theory provided the scientific community with the possibility of administering hormones, at least to
fetal animals, and subsequently observing the development of masculine
and feminine behavioral patterns. Nature provided Money and Ehrhardt
with humans in whom the prenatal hormonal effects could be investigated in terms of masculine or feminine behavior. According to Money
and Ehrhardt, "rapid advances in research from various disciplines have
opened new vistas against which to reexamine traditional behavioral
opinions on masculinity and femininity. . . . [We hope that] the theoretical
implications may serve as a focus of fruitful controversy. In connection
with the women's liberation movement they have, in fact, already engendered dispute."[35]

Money and Ehrhardt assumed an interactionist position within this
controversy. Nevertheless, in their book they strongly stressed the effects
of prenatal hormones on gender identity and the development of sexual
behavior.[36] Prenatal androgens and estrogens, male and female hormones, respectively, became metaphoric "boundary objects."[37] Money
and Ehrhardt's studies on the behavior of pseudohermaphrodites served
to delineate the domains of masculinity and femininity. Their descriptions
of the behavior of individuals whose brains were affected by abnormal
hormone levels revealed the characteristics of "natural" masculinity or
femininity in human behavior. Many viewed these descriptions as logical
truths.

A particular stimulus for acceptance of the organization hypothesis
was the theory's agreement with knowledge that had already been
accepted in the aforementioned fields: the sex-specific function of sex

hormones. According to this outlook, these chemicals were very suitable boundary objects for all work involving androgens and estrogens. They were both sufficiently elastic to adapt to local needs and the constraints of scientists in several disciplines and sufficiently robust in their function as "male" and "female" hormones to maintain a common identity across sites. Sex hormones acquired different meanings in different places, both inside and outside laboratory environments, although their structure was nevertheless common enough to more than one world to make them recognizable. In the early 1960s, endocrinologists and other scholars studying hormonal effects, such as hormonal influences on sex differentiation in the genitals and on brain differentiation, suggested a sex-specific function for gonadal hormones. Estrogens were often assigned to "the female sex hormones" and androgens to the "male sex hormones." Words such as "appropriate" or "heterotypical" were used to describe hormones, where "appropriate" signified androgens in males and estrogens in females, and "heterotypical" meant androgens in females and estrogens in males. Scientists considered androgens necessary for male development or functioning and estrogens and progesterone necessary for female development or functioning. Like many other researchers in the field, Richard Whalen, chair of the Department of Psychobiology of the University of California, Irvine, argued that in brain differentiation, the "applied hormone seemed to have an influence on the organization of the brain of mating behavior in the sense used by Young (1961) of producing changes in the responses to hormones different from those normally associated with an individual."[38]

Besides this sex-specific function, male and female hormones were thought to have opposing effects when administered to the other sex. Administering estrogen to a male rat, for example, would cause differentiation "in the opposite direction": it would "feminize" his brain. A "feminized" brain in this case entailed an increase in lordosis behavior. As the following passage illustrates, estrogens were seen as contrary and harmful to masculine behavior: "It is possible that estrogen treatment during infancy simply produces a functional castration, and that infantile castration leads to female-like behavior."[39]

It must be noted, however, that scientists in the 1960s could have been aware of reports on experiments, such as those performed in the 1930s as well as in the 1960s, which held that both androgens and estrogens had a masculinizing effect on behavior. Moreover, androgens and estrogens had been observed in both male and female organisms since the 1930s.[40] This information leads us to question why the sex-specific function of gonadal hormones became such a strong paradigm in biomedical research during the 1960s. In research, androgens were viewed as the sole agents responsible for masculinization and suppression of femininity in the brain, rather than *either* androgens *or* estrogens, as suggested by findings from the 1930s. Androgens and estrogens were clearly seen as carriers of biological maleness and femaleness, respectively.[41] This idea prevailed not only in neuroendocrinology, but throughout all disciplines concerned with the concept of sex hormones. The consensus among scientists that gonadal hormones served a dualistic function must be considered a condition for the acceptance of the organization theory.

Another reason for the acceptance of the organization hypothesis was its creation of a new domain of research that investigated groups of questions that had long gone unanswered. What kinds of research questions did this theory elicit? Judging from titles of articles published on the subject of sex differentiation in the brain in the journal *Hormones and Behavior* in the 1960s and 1970s, testing the masculinizing effects of different androgens in female rats became very popular.[42] The organization hypothesis offered an opportunity for investigating "masculinization" and the development of male sexual behavior. As this hypothesis held that fetal female rats did not have androgens, their brains were characterized as "undifferentiated."

In 1971, Roger Gorski, chair of the Department of Anatomy and Laboratory of Neuroendocrinology of the Brain at the UCLA School of Medicine, one of the most renowned research institutions concerned with brain differentiation, interpreted the organization theory as follows: "the concept of sexual brain differentiation postulates that the male rat secretes androgens to 'masculinize' his female brain."[43] Gorski's research focused less on brain differentiation in the sense of how brains became male or female than on the process for establishing male sexual behavior. Male sexual behavior was thought to originate in the androgens produced by the testes: "In order to produce a female model most representative of male physiology, we sought a level of androgen which would possibly mimic the action of the testes in the male."[44] Development of female sexual behavior was not investigated until the mid–1970s.[45]

Unlike earlier research with regard to the organization hypothesis, scientists began to experiment with the *permanent* prenatal effects of hormones. Before the proposal of the organization hypothesis, hormones were thought to have a *temporary* effect on the behavior of adult animals. The proposed hypothesis suggested that a permanent biological background for sexual behavior was created before birth. We may wonder about the reasons for the new popularity of research into the biological background of male sexual behavior and sexual behavior in general. Professor Jacob van der Werff ten Bosch, an endocrinologist at Erasmus University in Rotterdam who was involved in research on hormones and brain development in the 1960s, has given a clear reply to this question. According to van der Werff ten Bosch, the organization theory provided the answer to the world's preoccupation with homosexuality in the 1960s.[46] Both contemporary and earlier scientific research investigated the possibility of a hormonal cause for homosexuality. Despite measurements of hormone levels in urine, blood, and semen of homosexual men, no data were found to substantiate the assertion that homosexuality resulted from abnormal hormone levels.[47]

Comparing the organization theory with the theory of differentiation of the genital tract revealed that the genital tract differentiation theory explained the phenomenon of intersexes. Until that time, the socially contested occurrences of male and female homosexuality were viewed as "intersexuality in behavior." Men with a sexual preference for men were regarded as having a female sexual orientation, and lesbians were thought to have a male sexual orientation.[48] These phenomena could not be ascribed to the influence of temporary hormonal effects in adults. The organization theory promised a biological explanation for the development of masculine and feminine behavior in general and for the occurrence of homosexuality and lesbianism in particular. Biomedical scientists, who were concerned with hormonal effects, and psychologists and psychiatrists, who were concerned with behavior, joined forces in elucidating homosexuality and lesbianism by means of the organization theory. Illustrative of this argument is a passage from a paper presented at a symposium for psychiatrists on sexual deviation in 1983: "The elucidation of the interactions of intrauterine testosterone and its products with the foetal brain and neurotransmitters, [have] given us new models to understand the programming of sexuality."[49]

The final reason for the acceptance of the organization theory relates to the status of a particular discipline. We have already mentioned Frank Beach, who held different views about the origin of sex differences in behavior and did not subscribe to the theory and the ideas of Money and Ehrhardt, who extended the theory to include human behavior. Beach, a psychologist often regarded as the father of research into the relationship between hormones and behavior, believed that sexual behavior was rooted in the sensitivity of the genital organs and should be seen as the outcome of pleasurable sexual experience rather than as the outcome of differentiation of the brain. In his ironic article of 1971 he stated that "facts and laws pertaining to behavior stood in no need of 'validation' by correlating behavioral and neurophysiological phenomena . . . most students of behavior always have and always will derive a feeling of security and superiority that purport to 'explain' behavior in terms of known or imagined 'circuits', 'centers', or 'mechanisms' having a permanent address somewhere in the nervous system." Beach's next statement put the organization theory into perspective: "actually nearly all such 'mechanisms' consist of hypothetical constructs. . . ." The article concludes by proposing a close look at the "healthy trees" that would remain in the research after "our slash-and-burn treatment . . . reduces to ashes the more fragile and flammable saplings, bushes, and ferns which stood for unproven and tenuous speculations regarding connections between neurontogeny and adult behavior."[50]

The strong terms in which Beach stated his case may indicate that he felt his authority as a psychologist was at stake. The claims of biologists that hormones were the originators of animal and human behavior were detracting from the authority of psychologists, as exemplified by the assertions of Phoenix and his colleagues in their 1959 article (see above). Beach dissociated himself from the supporters of the organization theory with the following statement: "many theorists are so sadly and seriously afflicted with neurophilia (which in its terminal phases inevitably develops into cerebromania) that they are able seriously to entertain only those interpretations of behavior which are couched in the vocabulary of the neurologist . . . rather [I am] powerfully convinced by the behavioral evidence itself."[51]

In his 1971 article, Beach submitted an alternative model: he assumed that the undifferentiated brain was bisexual. This opinion differed from the presupposition of the architects of the organization theory, who saw the brain as inherently female at birth. In Beach's model, several types of hormones served a function, not just androgens. He argued that the opinion he had formed on this matter as far back as 1945 came closer to the "truth": "the sex hormones are best regarded not as stimuli or as organizing agents but as chemical sensitizers which alter the stimulability of critical mechanisms within the central nervous system."[52] At a conference in 1973, this argument was simplified and accentuated when Beach cried out during the discussion, "all is in the penis!" Gorski shouted "no, all is in the brain!"[53]

Beach challenged three of the organization theory's main claims. One of his points of criticism held that experimental evidence had proved unnecessary for treating newborn rats with androgen to depress or eliminate their subsequent displays of receptive behavior; Beach believed that the same results could be achieved by injecting young animals with estradiol during the sensitive period. He quoted several publications of the mid–1960s that mentioned this result.

In 1975, however, notwithstanding his severe criticism from four years earlier, Beach expressed limited agreement with the organization theory: "It is possible that normally occurring hormonal variations in the prenatal environment may have lifelong effects upon the behavioral response to hormones."[54] Beach made this statement after referring to Money and Ehrhardt's studies on prenatal hormone effects in humans. Apparently, he feared that he would otherwise lose his authority as a psychologist with stated assertions about the brain, hormones, and behavior. This retraction by unbeliever Frank Beach elevated the organization theory above any doubt among psychologists as well as among biologists.

As a psychologist, Beach argued with biomedical scientists. The psychologists Money and Ehrhardt rejected the feminist argument that genes are not at fault for the difference between the positions of women and men in society. Feminists have claimed that social environment is responsible for differences in behavior between women and men.[55] Money and Ehrhardt's shift from a genetic to a prenatal hormonal explanation for sex differences in behavior represents the response from the biomedical sciences to the feminist argument. Nevertheless, Money and Ehrhardt took the feminists' argument into account and did not completely overrule their claim. They called themselves "interactionists": they believed that both environment and biology are important factors in the explanation of differences between women and men. Most feminists were not very pleased with the outcome of the "negotiations about knowledge," as Ann Oakley called these exchanges: "From the emphasis on cultural factors evident in the 1950s and 1960s, we have moved through the middle ground of an interactionist line back towards outright biological determinism."[56]

Money and Ehrhardt were not concerned that feminists objected to their interactionism: their claims appeared to stand on very firm ground, and their book became a classic. They firmly established their authority as psychologists by making allegations regarding biomedical knowledge in the domain of human behavior. Both for Beach and for Money and Ehrhardt, the theory of the development of the male and female brain emerged as the victor.

The above reasons for the acceptance of the organization theory can be divided into scientific-philosophical factors, rooted in cultural images of masculinity and femininity, and reasons not directly rooted in these images. An example of the indirect basis is the need of several disciplines for a theory of the effects of hormones on behavior. Another source of the popularity of a theory that derives its direct basis from thought on masculinity and femininity was its facilitation of claims about permanent rather than temporary effects of hormones.

Questions related to masculinity and femininity have influenced the development of new domains of research for investigating old, unresolved issues concerning homosexuality. In all the disciplines mentioned, ideas about masculinity and femininity also affected generally accepted knowledge about the dualistic function ascribed to sex hormones: masculinity (in the brain) was seen as the result of "male" hormones, whereas femininity (in the brain) was attributed to the absence of the "Adam Principle," which was also referred to as the testes factor (i.e., androgens). This interpretation enabled the theory to fit smoothly into the existing dual image of gender, which emphasized Freud's idea that masculinity was the presence of a penis and femininity was the lack of a penis. The organization theory defined masculinity as the presence of male hormones, resulting in sexual initiative, action, intelligence, and an interest in a career, while femininity entailed an absence of male hormones, resulting in sexual receptiveness, passivity, a preoccupation with pretty clothes, and motherhood.[57] The functions of "male" and "female" hormones were scientific translations of perceptions of masculine and feminine behavior. The durability of the boundary function of "male" and "female" hormones will be demonstrated by the fates of scientific thought following the revelation of the need for converting "male" hormones into "female" hormones before "masculinizing" the brain.

Conversion of Androgens to Estradiol

As we saw, the dualistic function of gonadal hormones in the organization theory was a major factor in its acceptance by the scientific community. I will discuss the fate of a modification to the organization theory that did *not* accord with established views of the dual role of hormones. My description begins with the resistance to this modification among professional researchers.

In 1970, a group of scientists led by P. McDonald of the Department of Physiology at the Royal Veterinary College in London speculated that the actions of androgens in the brain were mediated by their metabolic conversion to estrogen.[58] Another group, led by Frederic Naftolin and Kenneth J. Ryan, who worked at the Department of Obstetrics and Gynecology at the University of California, San Diego, found metabolic conversion (also called aromatization) in the human fetus and started to look for the same process in the central nervous systems of rats.[59] Naftolin and Ryan seemed convinced of this conversion and immediately designated it as a concept. Other scientists, however, rejected their claim.[60] To explain the resistance by the field of research to the conversion hypothesis, a more detailed discussion of the reactions is in order.

Significantly, scientists were aware of the close similarity between the chemical structures of estradiol and testosterone. In the 1930s scientists found that both androgens and estrogens had the same effect on a rat's sex life. Moreover, when the organization theory was first proposed in 1959, it was argued that the masculinizing effect could be provoked by "testosterone or some metabolite." Estradiol is a metabolite of testosterone. Recalling the problem arising from Beach's critique of the function of hormones shows that the conversion theory accounted for all these factors. Scientists could therefore have been expected to respond with enthusiasm. Their reactions, however, were quite mixed and ranged from cautious acceptance to skepticism and from discountenance to amazement. A 1974 passage from Whalen is illustrative:

> This hypothesis is intriguing because it has been known since our early work that the administration of estrogen to newborn female rats will work like testosterone to inhibit the later display of lordosis behavior. . . . Of course, these findings in no way prove that sexual differentiation is controlled by an estrogen. The data are cited to raise the critical issue of the role of steroid metabolism in the differentiation process.[61]

Various articles argued that some androgen actions could be *mimicked* by estrogens, as if estrogens were incapable of operating as independent agents for masculinization. The hypothesis was also considered unable to account for effects of androgens on all neurobiological and neuro–behavioral systems. In the 1970s, scientists eagerly sought support for this claim.

In 1979, nine years after the first publication on this subject, Gorski appeared to accept the role of estradiol in masculinization: "we have the seemingly unusual situation where estradiol appears to be the vehicle for masculinization of the brain."[62] As late as 1984, however, the conversion hypothesis was clearly not regarded as a logical development in the field of brain differentiation: "Perhaps the most surprising is that estradiol mimics the differentiating effects of testosterone."[63] By then, some fifteen years later, the modification was accepted. Nevertheless, scientists' astonishment can still be registered in a statement such as the following: "Of particular fascination has been the discovery that estrogen, the potent female sex hormone, normally masculinizes the differentiating rat brain."[64]

Since the mid–1970s, this dual perception that biological masculinity and femininity are shaped by androgens and estrogens, respectively, has stubbornly persisted in neuroendocrinology and related fields. In recent (1992) text books of my students I found sex hormones indicated as male and female hormones; also, the terms "heterotypical" (androgens in females and estrogens in males) and "homotypical" (androgens in males and estrogens in females) are still in use. Even now in their lectures many scientists still explain their results by referring to male and female hormones. I came across a 1985 article by Whalen demonstrating that he had become aware of this phenomenon. Whalen argued:

> Testosterone is the most potent natural androgen known for maintaining sexual behavior in castrated males and in many species. But testosterone can also induce those responses characteristic of sexual receptivity in castrated females of several species. . . . These observations suggest that our attribution of a quality of a compound (e.g. defining testosterone as an androgen and not as an estrogen) *reflects an often unstated conviction about mechanism of action.*[65]

If we consider the problems researchers had in accepting "female" hormones as actually responsible for "masculinizing" the brain, we do not have to be surprised that mechanisms were constructed that ensured the unabated responsibility of androgens for male brain differentiation, thus ensuring the survival of the dualistic image of biological masculinity and femininity, translated into male and female hormones.

Mechanisms Perpetuating the Dual Function of Hormones

Had scientists been able to prove that estrogens originated exclusively from the conversion of circulating androgens, the conversion theory might have been accepted. In that case, scientists would have attributed male or female differentiations in the brain at birth to the respective presence or absence of androgens in the fetus, and the essence of the organization theory would have remained intact. In 1975, however, scientists discovered high levels of estrogens in the circulation of female rats during the period of brain differentiation.[66] They reported the same finding for male rats.[67] Scientists also found very high estrogen levels in primate fetuses during pregnancy. They speculated that this "female" hormone did not originate from the male fetus, but from the mother.[68] Consequently, urgent questions arose concerning the process for preventing masculinization of the brain of a female fetus.[69]

Investigators studying brain differentiation solved this mystery. They found that a protein circulating in fetal and neonatal animals was responsible for binding estrogens rather than androgens. This alpha fetoprotein, as it was called, was believed capable of binding the estradiol molecules; the resulting particle would be too big to pass through the barrier between the blood stream and the brain, whereas androgens, which they believed were not attracted to this protein, could reach the male brain. The conversion of these androgens into estradiol caused their masculinizing effect.[70] Their findings appeared to uphold the essence of the idea that androgens were responsible for masculine development.

In 1978, however, Klaus Döhler, who worked at the Department of Clinical Endocrinology of the Medical School in Hanover, Federal Republic of Germany, questioned the protective function of the alpha fetoprotein for estrogens. Döhler discussed the role of the protein and suggested that instead of creating a protective barrier against estrogens, alpha fetoprotein mediated the transport of estrogens into the target cell.[71] Scientists had indeed reported finding some of this alpha fetoprotein inside brain cells in that year.[72] This discovery meant that a different answer was necessary to safeguard the belief that testosterone (androgen) was responsible for the masculinization of the brain.

A new solution was found in the differentiation of estrogen and androgen receptors in brain cells. These receptors were reportedly located in different parts of the brain and could be detected during different periods that coincided with the masculinizing process of sexual differentiation in the brains of the rats.[73] This solution ensured that males were born with "male" brains and females with "female" brains. Again, the dualistic idea of hormonal effects on brain differentiation survived, and the modification of the organization theory was accepted.

Conclusions

Evaluating the development of neuroendocrinological research in the last three decades reveals the powerful influence of dualistic thought about masculinity and femininity, translated into dualistic effects of hormones. These views have determined the acceptability of a theory. In comparing the acceptance of the organization theory with the acceptance of the conversion theory, we have seen that the organization theory was accepted and extended to nonsexual types of behavior within five years after it was proposed, whereas the conversion theory was accepted only after ample mechanisms were constructed to ensure that principles concerning the dual effects of hormones were upheld. Initially, dualistic thought regarding gonadal hormones impeded the acceptance of the conversion theory.

Moreover, the dualistic beliefs about masculinity and femininity that prevailed in western society during the 1960s, which were manifested in the dualistic role ascribed to gonadal hormones, determined the course that research was allowed to take. The dualism of the organization theory stood in the way of research on issues concerning the development of female sexual behavior, as such behavior was merely considered the effect of an absence of androgens. Female sexual behavior was not deemed subject to manipulation by hormones; if hormones were administered, sexual behavior would necessarily be "masculinized" and would thus become part of research on the development of male sexual behavior. Female sexual behavior was viewed only as a response to being mounted by a male. In the 1960s, therefore, research based on the organization theory was permitted to focus only on elucidating the development of male heterosexual and homosexual behavior. Investigation of the development and nature of female sexual behavior was neglected until the late 1970s; in the early 1970s, research addressed the process of preventing the masculinization of "female" brains.

Dualistic thought about masculinity and femininity has led to the belief that male and female brains are essentially different—probably as a response to the need for a biological theory explaining the differences in the social functioning of men and women. Prior to the organization theory, no valid "scientific" theory existed that based these differences on biological aspects of the brain. Scientists believed that the variations in behavior between men and women were caused by androgens that resulted in sexual initiative, activity, aggression, and intelligence in males. These characteristics were considered undeveloped (or far less developed) in females because of the absence of androgens before birth. Nature was thought to predestine females to a lifetime of caring and social and sexual submission. In this context, the "hormonal" explanation provided by science for these features endowed the dualistic images of masculinity and femininity that existed in society with a scientific "truth." As Bleier, Fausto-Sterling, and Birke explained, the organization theory *reproduced* stereotypes of masculinity and femininity. Simultaneously, the theory *produced* the image that masculinity and femininity in behavior was based on biological sex differences within the brain. Bruno Latour has argued that images of subjects of scientific investigations can change, and that laboratory research can generate new images.[74] This assertion appears to be valid for research based on the organization theory with regard to the images of masculinity and femininity within the brain.

With respect to the "truth" suggested by these images around 1970, it cannot be overlooked that most scientists were men. Few women had professional careers, and women who were in a position to contribute to intellectual development in science were the exception. At that time, the image of femininity as contradictory to a career was plausible. We cannot ignore this situation in our efforts to understand the eager acceptance of the organization theory. The association by male scientists of androgens (male sex hormones) with masculinity and male gender identity in their adoption of the organization theory explains their difficulty with the idea that "female" hormones were important in the masculinization of the brain and the development of "male" behavior. The chemicals associated with masculinity and femininity were boundary objects, and it was hard to accept that these boundary objects did not respect the barriers between masculinity and femininity in intellectual or social respects. The next chapter relates the consequences that arose when women scientists crossed the threshold of the laboratory despite such preconceptions in the early 1970s.

3

FEMINISM AND THE BIOLOGICAL CONSTRUCTION OF FEMALE AND MALE BEHAVIOR

Introduction

The previous chapter compared the relatively smooth acceptance of the original organization theory within the scientific community to the reception of the modified version. The key to understanding this situation appeared to be the "masculinizing" function ascribed to androgens. Until the early 1970s, this field of research overlooked "feminizing" processes in brain and behavior in theoretical and experimental respects, and laboratories generally lacked female staff. Male scientists formulated the questions and designed the research methods. This state of affairs began to change during the 1970s. Women opted to pursue higher education and entered professional life and laboratory environments in increasing numbers. They contributed to research by visualizing phenomena that had remained invisible in research methods applied thus far; they became involved in "articulation work."[1] This development stimulated an emphasis on prenatal history in explanations for "dimorphism" in the behavior of males and females; behavior became sexualized in biological respects (see chap. 1, fig. 1.1).[2]

Throughout this period, the old nature versus nurture controversy haunted many disciplines[3] and provided feminists with a framework for questioning the origins of female behavior and sex differences. Although the full panoply of feminist perspectives still awaited a complete and recognizable articulation in the early 1970s, a few distinctive visions had appeared on the horizon.

Germaine Greer's argument against biological determinism represented the dominant position in feminism. According to Greer, biological sex differences cannot explain differences between male and female behavior and social inequalities between women and men. Rather, disparities are caused by education and other social factors.[4] Although a dissenting feminist minority believed in a female nature, not all proponents of this view embraced the biological explanations for the inequalities.[5] Mainstream feminists called their dissenting counterparts essentialists. In general, feminism either ignored biology or countered biological arguments with sociological explanations for sex differences in behavior.

Recently, Helen Longino, a feminist philosopher of science, argued that "as long as feminists counter biological explanations for behavioral differences with competing environmental explanations of their origin, masculinity and femininity are thought of as real elements of a dichotomy." Longino suggests that "though feminists' goal is overcoming gender dichotomization, this will reinforce as much as it will challenge the dichotomy of masculinity and femininity."[6] As we will see, gender dichotomization was indeed reinforced in the 1970s. Feminists, women scientists, and their male colleagues were all extremely interested in the origins of masculinity and femininity. Although their ideas differed about the nature of these origins, sex and gender dichotomization clearly resulted from the coconstruction of all parties interested in sex differences. I will describe the positions and entrenchments of the different participants and their impact on research in neuroendocrinology in terms of theoretical concepts, research methods, and results. Next, I will present the conditions that enabled feminist ideas to become integrated into science and that led feminists to join forces in constructing gender dichotomy and in challenging the dichotomy between masculinity and femininity.

Biological Theory of Development of Behavior

Man and Woman, Boy and Girl: Differentiation and Dimorphism of Gender Identity from Conception to Maturity by John Money and Anke A. Ehrhardt, which was published in 1972, discussed the effects of prenatal hormones on the behavior of adult humans and was the culmination of research about sexual behavior conducted on animal models that appeared to be equivalent to humans. The ideas can be traced back to the beginning of this century, when researchers started to ascribe differences in sexual behavior to the newly developed concept of sex hormones. In 1913, Steinach proposed that differences in gonadal hormones secreted by the testes or ovaries during adulthood provided a satisfactory explanation for all behavioral discrepancies between male and female adult rats.[7] At that time, scientists were experimenting with ovary implants in castrated male or testicular tissue in ovariectomized females. In 1919, Carl Moore, who had been extremely reluctant was to attribute behavior to hormone activity,[8] concluded: "These observations tend to support very strongly the ideas of the transforming power of the gonad of one sex over, at least, the psychic nature of the opposite sex."[9]

This passage implies an opposing relationship between a male and a female psychic nature. Moreover, scientists considered differences in behavior (psychic nature) between male and female animals to be fully explained by the presence of testes or ovaries. They believed these organs were responsible for producing sex-specific "male" and "female" hormones: essential chemical substances in the functioning of adult males or females. During the 1930s, however, scientists' assumptions concerning the origin and function of male and female hormones were challenged. In 1934, Bernard Zondek wrote a letter to *Nature* about an unexpected result: He had found a high concentration of female hormones in the urine of stallions. Until then, large quantities of female hormones had been measured in the urine of pregnant mares, whereas the excretion of female hormones by nonpregnant mares had been very small. In the same year, Zondek reported a result that was even more remarkable at that time. He had discovered an even richer source of female hormones in the testes of stallions than in their urine. By the late 1930s, scientists had begun to accept the conclusion that "male" and "female" hormones occurred and functioned in both sexes. After 1935, the function of sex hormones was no longer considered sex-specific, nor were the actual hormones exclusively associated with characteristics related to sex or viewed as antagonists. They were seen as chemicals that generated manifold synergistic actions in both the female and the male body. In the late 1930s, scientists changed the absolute sex-specific function of hormones to a relative sex-specific function by postulating that while both male and female hormones were important for the function of bodies of both sexes, female hormones served an additional purpose in female reproduction.[10]

As described in chapter 2, this relative sex specific function of sex hormones was abandoned in 1959, the year of the birth of the organization theory. Androgens and estrogens were restored to their roles as chemical messengers for masculinity and femininity, respectively. Charles Phoenix, Robert Goy, Arnold Gerall, and William Young, the founders of the organization theory, ascribed an important mechanism in sexual functioning to the male hypothalamus. According to their theory, the male hypothalamus (and male sexual behavior) developed in the presence of androgens before or around birth, depending on the species.[11] Scientists referred to male sexual behavior as mounting: One animal would climb onto another animal's back. In the absence of androgens, however, the hypothalamus would remain undifferentiated, and female sexual behavior (i.e., an arching of the back), called "lordosis" and regarded as a measure of receptivity, would result.[12] Although in most species, both sexes were known to exhibit the sexual behavior of the other sex, most topical publications from the 1960s neglected to elucidate the definition of certain behavior as masculine or feminine.

Scientists saw male behavior, unlike female behavior, as complex. In experimental situations they distinguished numerous components: mounting, intromission and ejaculation, and combinations of these acts. Female behavior was "objectified" in a different way from male behavior: Lordosis was unequivocally considered a measure of female receptivity to her male counterpart. Scientists defined the intensity of receptivity, a measure of female brain development (or rather nondevelopment, because this reaction was seen as basic), as the lordosis quotient (LQ): the number of times that an animal reacted with lordosis to being mounted by another animal. Thus, scientists perceived female sexual behavior simply as a response to a "male" mount. They did not register active female sexual behavior or passive male behavior. In fact, male and female behavior were considered to be opposites that corresponded to the functions of hormones in the brain as designated. The absence of androgens resulted in a female undifferentiated brain (the opposite of a male differentiated brain) and caused passivity or receptivity (the opposite of male sexual activity).

The theory had consequences for the scope of possible research topics. As active female sexual behavior did not exist within the framework of the organization theory in the 1960s, it was not studied; androgens and masculinity in the brain ruled the investigations of behavior.[13]

Masculinity and Femininity in the Experiments

How were scientists able to overlook active female contributions to sexual interactions in experiments? How did they match "male" hormones, male brain development, and masculinity in the behavior of laboratory rodents?

During the 1960s, the main question in most experiments was, "What makes a brain male?" In experiments, scientists focused on behavior that fit their definition of male nature and developed experimental designs that rendered female laboratory rodents' contributions to sexual interactions invisible. Examples from an article by Gorski, the director of one of the most important research institutes concerned with brain differentiation (the Department of Anatomy and Laboratory of Neuroendocrinology of the Brain of the UCLA School of Medicine), illustrate this process. In this article, which was published in 1971, he noted some problems in the field research and suggested that contradictory results could be explained by the testing procedure.[14] Other problems concerned scientists' different definitions of receptivity among laboratory rats.

In the 1960s, as Gorski described, male rats were generally allowed time to adjust to the testing arena when performing a behavioral test. Scientists found that males, removed from their home cage and placed in a test situation, did not respond until they had spent about two hours adapting to the new situation. After this adaptation period the test female was placed in the cage. Scientists then observed and quantified the behavior (times of mounting, intromission, and ejaculation) of the hormone-treated male in interaction with the "stimulus" female.[15] The quantity of male behavior was considered a measure of prenatal hormone action in masculinizing the rat's brain. In 1969, the results of an experiment were published that had involved testing "the possibility that a female rat is unusually sensitive to a novel environment." Scientists placed female rats who had received prenatal androgen treatments in the test arena for two hours before introducing a male. Gorski described how "under this testing condition most females exhibited a very high LQ."[16] He did not expect this result. According to the organization theory, the androgens should have "masculinized" the brains of these female rats, resulting in low receptivity, a low LQ.[17] While Gorski did not explain this unexpected occurrence, both female and male rats were clearly sensitive to novel environments. This approach is typical of scientists' attitudes toward females during the 1960s in that it reflects concern about the effects of adaptation on male sexual behavior but shows no regard for the effects on female sexual behavior.

The discussion about the different measures of sexual behavior also revealed that scientists espoused different views of male and female sexual behavior in experiments. Gorski stressed that a detailed analysis and proper definition of male behavior was essential for an adequate study of brain differentiation. Discrepancies between scientists' applications of the terms lordosis and receptivity, however, also gave rise to difficulties. Richard Whalen and Ronald Nadler stated: "Intromission and ejaculation by the males induced a forced arching of the back in the females which did not outlast the duration of the males' response. These responses might be termed 'forced lordosis responses,' and they can be easily discriminated from the typical lordosis of the receptive female."[18] Unlike Whalen and Nadler, Gorski, who treated females in the same way, considered them to be receptive. He used the presence of spermatozoa in the vagina as a definition of receptivity, though he considered this measure weaker than spontaneous lordosis.[19] Whalen and Nadler agreed that if receptivity is defined as spermatozoa in the vagina, the female rats were indeed receptive. To solve the problem of defining lordosis, Whalen and Nadler suggested distinguishing between forced intromission with a "passive or weakly receptive female" and mounts or intromissions accompanied by a normal lordosis response.

This struggle over definitions of the female role in the sexual interactions of rats and the experiments concerning adaptation time for female animals illustrate that researchers viewed female animals as instruments for investigating male sexual behavior. Over the years, some objections had been raised concerning the neglect of the female role in this field of research. Frank Beach's presentation of his criticism provides the most interesting insight into the evolution of these ideas.

Criticism of the Organization Theory

As I argued in the previous chapter, Frank Beach, a psychologist and authority on research on hormones and behavior, criticized the research based on the organization theory for brain development in an effort to persuade scientists in the field to abandon this theory of hormones for an approach based on psychological research.[20] This section relates his criticism to scientific thought about the role of hormones in the development of sexual behavior and considers the consequences of Beach's reproaches.

First, Beach noted the rigid attitude toward the differentiation of male and female behavior. He asserted that scientists in the 1960s had overlooked the possibility that animals could exhibit sexual behavior associated with the other sex, meaning that males and females could exhibit mounting as well as lordosis. Moreover, in the proposal of the theory in 1959, male and female behavior were regarded as tendencies in males and females rather than as behavior that was exclusive to either sex.[21] In this way, Beach provided the first criticism of the dual concepts of male and female sexual behavior and turned the attention of scientists to female behavior.

Beach also argued that both estrogen and androgen treatments had been observed to increase mounting behavior in females. Beach thus criticized the idea of the specificity of hormones in the organization theory. Most scientists, however, believed (and some even published results to this effect) that *if* estrogens had any effect on brain development, it would be the opposite to that of androgens. In males, estrogens were thought to cause an absence of copulation behavior rather than an augmentation of male sexual behavior.[22] Thus, Beach's article abandoned both the dual concepts of sexual behavior and the dualistic function of hormones. In his view estrogens could masculinize the brain as well as androgens.

Beach's third point of criticism was that prenatal hormones also affected the growth of the penis. In fact, Beach viewed androgens as "organizers" of the penis and as chemicals that affected its sensitivity and therefore sexual experiences as well. In the 1940s, he postulated that the lessons of these experiences contained the key to understanding the development of sexual behavior, rather than brain "organization."[23] A strong argument in support of his model surfaced when some researchers published the results of tests of male sexual behavior conducted on genetically male animals, which, due to early hormonal treatments, did not even have penises.[24] Beach had claimed that researchers had overlooked the possibility that the presence or absence of a penis affected behavior.

As described in the previous chapter, most scientists in the field took Beach's objections seriously but nevertheless adhered to the organization theory. A memorial published in 1988, the year that Beach died, referred to his critical article from 1971 as an "attempt to clarify the thinking of the many who were studying the sexual differentiation process and to ensure the logical construction of concepts and to provide guidance for their fruitful application."[25] One possible reading of this statement is that the authors of the memorial wanted to honor Beach for his valuable criticism and bury his failure to adhere to the organization theory.

If we compare the concepts of masculinity and femininity in behavior and the function of hormones as perceived by Beach with the roles attributed by the adherents of the organization theory, Beach's conception of the sexes appears less rigid. He considered male and female behavior possible for both sexes. Furthermore, the function Beach ascribed to "male" and "female" hormones was less dualistic than in most contemporary articles: Estrogens could play a role in masculinizing behavior. Beach's criticism put a dent in the stronghold of dualism in concepts of male and female behavior and the functions of hormones. On the other hand, it is striking that the essence in Beach's theory as well as in those of most other researchers regarding the development of sexual behavior involved a central "masculine" element. "Male" hormones originating from the testes or the sensitivity of the penis were crucial to understanding the development of sexual behavior. In 1971, the ideas of Beach and most other researchers accorded with Freud's philosophy, which considers the male sexual organ to be the origin of sexuality. Although Freud did not posit a simple correspondence between biology and psychology, he attributed universal psychic differences between the sexes to anatomical differences. Freud expressed doubts about the strict biological basis and normative character of his observations, but ultimately assumed that the female's lack of a penis condemned her to biological and psychological inferiority. Without a penis, she was unable to develop into a mature, autonomous, and rational individual.[26] Beach differed from the adherents of the organization theory in the importance he attached to the penis, while the others located the center for sexual behavior in the brain. Both parties reproduced a one-sided male heterosexual vision[27] on sexuality. In experiments with male hormones, development of either male brains or penis was matched with masculine behavior by circular reasoning that excluded all aspects of femininity. Important for the following section is that Beach was the only scientist who dissented with the organization theory in this field of research. Soon we will see how he developed this view.

A Cry for the Liberation of the Female Rodent

The neglect of female sexual behavior in scientific research had always been a source of criticism. Gordon Bermant, a psychologist who worked with laboratory rats, and John Calhoun, an ethologist who studied wild rats, remarked on the one-sided interest in male sexual behavior.[28] In the 1960s, scientists involved in biological research into prenatal hormone effects on male brain development clearly ignored these comments. By the second half of the 1970s, the women's movement managed to open up the masculine circle to include femininity. Who achieved this feat, and what was their motivation? What were the consequences?

As a result of the women's movement, more women opted to pursue higher education and to enter the field of behavioral neuroendocrinology. Some of these women provided historical contributions to this discipline. In 1970, Monica Schoelch-Krieger, a biology researcher at Rutgers University, lectured at a conference about an experiment in which she tied down male rats and gave female rats the opportunity to react to the tied males. Her video demonstrated behavior that had previously been invisible to those present at the conference.[29] To their amazement, the viewers witnessed the female rats display a comprehensive repertoire of sexual behavior, of which lordosis was only one element.[30] After this conference, female sexual behavior became an increasingly popular subject of investigation among both female and male researchers. For example, Bengt Meyerson and L. H. Lindström at the Department of Pharmacology of the University of Uppsala in Sweden published an article on a methodology for studying sexual *motivation* among females.[31] In 1972, the Czech scientists Jaroslav Madlafousek and Zdenek Hlinak published a paper about the *appetitive* or *precopulatory* sexual behavior of female rats.[32] In addition, investigators of primate behavior explicitly stressed the need to distinguish between "some parameters which reflect *initiation* of sexual interaction by the female," and those "in which the female allows interaction initiated by the male."[33] By the 1970s, such remarks no longer fell on deaf ears but stimulated other researchers to think about their investigations.

In 1974, Richard Doty, a postdoctoral researcher in psychology who was studying hormonal effects on animal behavior at the same institute as Beach, published an article entitled: "A Cry for the Liberation of the Female Rodent: Courtship and Copulation in Rodentia,"[34] in which he argued that the "behavior of the female has been ignored in most studies of rodent copulation." Doty attributed this imbalance to a number of interacting factors. The first reason he mentioned was that investigators of behavior studied male rodent behavior with the traditional objective of ultimately formulating monolithic laws of behavior intended for general application to most members of the animal kingdom, including females. Second, he found that most experiments on sexual behavior studied copulation in small and confined test situations in which the male appeared more dominant and active than the female. He argued that the earlier phases of courtship, which feature mate selection, pair formation, and other conduct related to sexual behavior, had not been examined. Doty also explained that the male's copulatory behavior was more obvious than the female's and could easily be divided into components that were sensitive to a number of experimental manipulations in laboratory studies. Doty's third argument was that the estrous cycle of females affected some of the hormonal and behavioral variables used by scientists and was a general nuisance for many investigators.

According to Doty, male subjects were overrepresented numerically, and conclusions drawn from experiments with males were more likely to be overgeneralized than conclusions from tests done on females. He noted the importance of investigations of female sex initiation and quoted extensively from Calhoun's study (published twelve years earlier) on sexual behavior among wild rats and its complexity in both males and females, in addition to the nonbehavioral aspects of, for example, odor spreading and sounds.[35] Doty argued that rats used for laboratory experiments were inbred in comparison to their wild counterparts and suggested that this characteristic affected their behavior.[36] He concluded that laboratory studies could oversimplify the complexity of sexual behavior in most natural situations. In conclusion, he expressed the hope "that the present article will extend the interests of many behaviorists to courtship phenomena in wild species and will stimulate more 'equal opportunity' research on female rodents."[37]

Doty's title "A Cry for the Liberation of the Female Rodent," as well as the words "equal opportunity" in the concluding sentence were slogans of the women's liberation movement at the end of the 1960s and the beginning of the 1970s.[38] These terms were clearly convincing rhetoric, and soon the subject of female sexual behavior resulted in the proposal of new concepts.

In 1975, Frank Beach responded to this new development. He asked: "Why had there been so much interest in male copulation and so little interest in the female part of sexual behavior?" He mentioned that "this [was] often neglected, especially by male investigators and theorists."[39] In an article from 1976, Beach argued that the "female's tendency to display appetitive responses finds little opportunity for expression in laboratory experiments which focus exclusively upon her receptive behavior, or upon the male's execution of his coital pattern. The resulting concept of essentially passive females receiving sexually aggressive males seriously misrepresents the normal mating sequence and encourages a biased concept of feminine sexuality. Failure to recognize the importance of female initiative in the mating of laboratory rodents has been noted."[40] His article was designed to "propose certain correctives for the existing imbalance and, at the same time, attempt[ed] to provide a simple but heuristically useful scheme with theoretical and practical implications for the study of feminine sexuality and its behavioral expression."[41] Beach was referring to the studies of Richard Doty and the other studies mentioned above. In fact, his article served as a theoretical convergence of the different concepts that had been developed at the beginning of the 1970s, for example, consummatory or appetitive behavior, or sexual motivation of female rats.

Beach proposed dividing female sexual behavior into attractivity, proceptivity, and receptivity. He provided the three basic concepts with operational definitions in terms of stimulus-response relationships that were suitable for quantitative measurement.

This article became a classic among accounts of studies on hormonal effects on brain development and behavior, both because of the new concepts and because of Beach's final acceptance of the organization theory. Beach did not, however, subscribe to the theory in its traditional version but modified it to reflect his former beliefs. Previously, he had denied that the brain was inherently female and argued that several types of hormones could serve as "chemical sensitizers." Now, Beach relocated the activity of these "chemical sensitizers" from the sexual organs in adulthood to prenatal brains in both males and females.

At the end of Beach's article he assumed that different parts of the brain in both males and females were responsible for the different types of behavior distinguished in his model. He considered estrogens especially important in the prenatal female brain. This view is surprising, since his references dealt with hormone effects in adulthood. If Beach's sole intention was to propose new concepts for studying active female sexual behavior, he need not have addressed the prenatal hormone paradigm. After the publication of his 1971 article, however, Beach had become rather isolated from his colleagues because he did not adhere to the prenatal hormone paradigm. In 1976, his subscription to the organization theory enabled him to resume discussions with colleagues in the field who did not doubt the theory's validity.

Beach's article had important consequences for the study of female sexual behavior and for the localization of the control mechanisms that scientists ascribed to it. In the years that followed, many researchers, including many women such as Martha McClintock, Donna Emery, Mary Erskine, Anne Etgen, Francien de Jonge, Kathie Olsen, Jane Stewart, and Christina Williams focused on female sexual behavior in animals.[42] Following Beach's hypothesis, some studied the parts of the brain that regulated the expression of proceptive or solicitation behavior. The most suitable candidates for investigating neuroendocrine regulation of female sexual behavior were various parts of the hypothalamus, which were thought to be involved in reproduction.[43] Scientists investigated the control mechanism of female sexual behavior in this part of the brain by making lesions in and by affecting different parts of rat hypothalami with chemicals (naloxone, beta-endorphine, or steroid hormone implants).[44] Now the interest in the sexual behavior of female rats led to investigations that caused brain damage in the subject. Prior to Beach's article female rats were subjected only to hormone injections and ovariectomy.[45]

Reinventing Female Appetitive Activities

Let us take a closer look at the new concepts that Beach proposed and examine the stimulus his work gave to redressing the existing imbalance. How did his female colleagues appreciate the innovation?

Beach defined the new concept of *attractivity* for females as "her stimulus value to the sexual performance of a male of the same species, or, the female's capacity to elicit ejaculation." In descriptions, attractivity covers the full range of stimulation including bringing a male to a female, assisting males in identifying the female's sex and reproductive status, synchronizing and orienting the male's coital responses, and finally, promoting the emission of sperm while the penis is in the vagina.[46] Thus, definitions and descriptions both associated female attractivity with male sexual behavior and copulation.

Given the period of attractivity and the hormones thought to be involved, scientists obviously considered *reproduction* the ultimate goal for female animals.[47] According to Beach, attractivity was positively affected by estrogens and negatively by progesterone. Progesterone was assumed to be produced at the end of the reproductive period (when females are not fertile), and estrogens were produced in high levels during estrus or ovulation (when females are fertile). Beach perceived attractivity as helpful to the reproductive capacity of females and as essential to the survival of the species since "it maximizes the probability of copulation when the female is fertile and susceptible to impregnation."

Beach proposed *proceptivity* as a basis for investigating the sexual initiative of female animals: "Appetitive activities shown by females in response to stimuli received from males" or "proceptive responses are parameters which reflect initiation of sexual interaction by the female."[48] These definitions left little opportunity for female initiative in sexual behavior. Beach used the term "response" in the definition of proceptivity or in the defined behavior. The function of proceptivity, a bit similar to that of attractivity was "to intensify the males' sexual excitement, when this is necessary, and also to facilitate, coordinate and synchronize the bodily adjustments necessary for genital union and penile insertion." Thus, proceptivity is also seen as behavior that facilitates copulation. The addition of "when this is necessary" after "to intensify the male's sexual excitement" is remarkable. Nevertheless, Beach added another function to proceptivity, not primarily oriented to copulation but to the female animal herself: "to increase the level of excitement in the performing female. And although no systematic studies of this effect appears in the literature, its occurrence is intuitively apparent to experienced observers and deserves direct examination."[49] In describing the experiments of other scientists on proceptivity, however, he applied the first function of proceptivity. Proceptivity is described as: (1) the tendency of females to approach and remain in the vicinity of males, (2) invitation behavior, such as making special gestures and vocalizing, and (3) the mounting of a male by a female is considered proceptive behavior.

Proceptivity was thought to be stimulated by different hormones. According to Beach, proceptivity, like attractivity, occurred solely or more frequently (depending on the species) at the time of ovulation of the female animal and was positively affected by high levels of estrogens. Other scientists, however, claimed that female "motivation" or proceptivity was augmented following androgen treatments ("male" hormones).[50] Clinical literature identified testosterone as the "libido hormone" in women.[51] In his reference to a clinical study, Beach implicitly compared rats' proceptivity to women's libido.

On the level of the functioning of hormones, scientists found it difficult to designate "female" hormones as agents in the display of sexual initiative, which was traditionally considered a male activity. Beach tried to solve the problem by suggesting the "possibility that testosterone is converted to estrogen before it produces effects on the behavior of female monkeys and rats."[52]

Though Beach's definitions did not fully liberate the sexual life of female rats, they helped correct the imbalance in knowledge about female sexual behavior. The 1970s marked the beginning of ascribing sexual activity to female animals and to investigating this behavior. To what extent did Beach redress the imbalance about male sexual behavior? Were males now also considered capable of receptivity? And could "female" hormones be assigned a function in male sexual behavior?

According to Beach, *receptivity* is "distinguished by the ubiquity of its usage and the infrequency of definition . . . and if undefined terms were employed with the implicit assumption of mutual understanding, the outcome could be utter confusion." In Beach's opinion, receptivity "constitutes the consummatory phase of the mating sequence, but there is no hard and fast separation between consummatory and appetitive aspects of sexual interaction." Moreover, since for the "majority of mammals, reception of the male *in copulo* involves much more than immobile acquiescence by the female, active cooperation may be essential to successful mating."[53] Although Beach changed the definition and the meaning of receptivity from passive to active, this behavior continued to be registered only in females.

Why did he describe it that way? Let us examine the following example provided by Beach. In the case of male gorillas, who "rarely attempt to copulate unless the female initiates sexual interaction,"[54] the male is not designated as receptive. This passage in Beach's article served to illustrate female proceptive behavior. Receptivity apparently remained reserved for animals that could accommodate a penis. Beach thus introduced a more balanced explanation for female sexual behavior by proposing new concepts. Nevertheless, the approach to studying male sexual behavior remained unchanged.

The period of receptivity and the function of the hormones that stimulated receptivity also stayed the same: "Successful mating and the chance of conception is the highest during the period in which the level of estrogens is high, around ovulation." Female hormones were not assigned a role in sexual functioning of males, although some researchers found that androgens could increase receptivity among female monkeys.[55] While Beach quoted this experiment in his article, he also argued that "variability of receptivity in period of occurrence in the order of primates is great and the range of species examined so limited that generalizations regarding hormonal effects on primate receptivity are highly speculative." His reasoning might have become entangled in the function of hormones in sexual and reproductive behavior: Sexual behavior was seen as "male" and thus needed androgens, and reproductive behavior was regarded as "female" and thus required estrogens. In any case, little changed in the study of male sexual behavior. Neither male receptivity nor the function of estrogens in male sexual behavior were questioned.

Beach did, however, succeed in proposing "certain correctives for the existing imbalance" in 1976. How did other researchers view this field? Also in 1976, Beach's former students presented papers in honor of his sixty-fifth birthday. Leonore Tiefer, the only woman in his program, presented a paper entitled: "The Context and Consequences of Contemporary Sex Research: A Feminist Analysis."[56] Tiefer revealed her view that giving females the opportunity to demonstrate their appetitive activities was only a small step toward a better understanding of sexual interactions. She argued that considerations of female sexual behavior, male reproductive physiology, the subjective aspects of sexuality, and the nonerotic components of sexuality had been impoverished, both by excessive reliance on one rigid scientific model and by using the masculine experience as the primary point of reference. She concluded with suggestions "toward a non-sexist understanding of human sexuality." How did Beach react? Tiefer later wrote: "Frank was horrified by my critique, and I remember him raving loudly about how anti-scientific thinking like mine would have ruinous, simply ruinous, consequences."[57] Beach's use of the term antiscientific shows the true meaning of "articulation work."[58] As Tiefer's arguments covered matters that had clearly been "invisible" until then, her criticism did not fit into rationalized models of scientific investigation. Moreover, Beach had already contributed to the repair of part of the "imbalance" and clearly was not ready to accept feminist criticism again from a student. This makes "articulation work" in science a hard job. Tiefer had the courage not to give up, even though this incident affected her deeply. In a paper written in 1992, in which she reminisces about the incident, she repeats her criticism as formulated in 1976 (which was obviously in need of being repeated).[59] In 1988, she received an award for her 1976 paper from the Association for Women in Psychology.

Tiefer's criticism mainly concerned the study of human sexual behavior. How is the correction of the imbalance perceived in studies of sexual behavior in animals? Mary Erskine, now Research Associate Professor at the Department of Biology at Boston University, who pursued the findings of Schoelch-Krieger and other female researchers, wrote: "Our ideas about what makes up feminine sexual responsiveness have been influenced by the preconceptions drawn from work on males. The male viewpoint: i.e. 'attractivity' and 'proceptivity' are measured and defined by the responses that the *male makes to the female,* not by the behavior patterns displayed by the female herself. Therefore, even the language used to describe female sexual behavior is biased toward the male perspective."[60]

Notwithstanding the remaining criticism, the intellectual changes of the 1970s had sweeping consequences. While until 1976 most scientists had seen receptivity as a product of undifferentiated brains, they now accepted Beach's suggestion that "proceptive and receptive behavior may depend upon different anatomical or neuro-chemical systems in the brain."[61] The transformation in scientific concepts due to the entrance of women scientists in laboratories and Beach's subscription to the organization theory resulted in the expansion of ideas about the role of prenatal hormones in the brain to include the "second sex." Following this development, the prenatal hormone paradigm of brain development grew stronger than ever before in the second half of the 1970s. This situation greatly affected both scientists' and feminist scientists' perceptions of sex differences in human behavior.

Feminism and the Biological Construction of Human Behavior

What consequences did the prenatal hormone paradigm have for investigations of male and female behavior in humans in the 1970s? Previously, the application of the prenatal hormone paradigm in humans served mainly to elucidate the development of male sexual behavior. The ideas of Dörner, who used this understanding in his attempts to prevent or cure male homosexuality, were controversial in this field of research.[62] During the late 1960s and 1970s, feminism caused scientists to shift their interest toward sex differences; the prenatal hormone paradigm became popular in all disciplines involved in studies of human behavior.

As described in the previous chapter, Money and Ehrhardt were the first to consider behavioral categories other than sexual behavior, but nevertheless associated behavior with masculinity and femininity within the paradigm of prenatal hormones. The publication of their book, *Man and Woman, Boy and Girl,* marked the culmination of the development of ideas about sex, which had been studied in animal models and were thought to be equivalent in humans. As in animal research, Money and Ehrhardt believed prenatal androgens caused "activity" in humans, defined as outdoor vigor, athletic abilities, body contact sports, and kinesis. Androgens also affected dress habits (called unisex in the case of practical clothes for girls), career ambitions, and high IQs. Other behavioral categories were thought to result from the *absence* of androgens and were associated with femininity: fantasies about motherhood, playing with dolls, preferences for pretty dresses, and lower IQs.[63] Although Money and Ehrhardt later withdrew their claim that IQ and sexual orientation were affected by androgens, many other researchers continued this line of research. Money and Ehrhardt's later work reflected greater subtlety and caution in the conclusions about prenatal hormone effects on "sex dimorphic behavior."[64]

Following Money and Ehrhardt, researchers in several disciplines investigated countless behavioral variables associated with masculinity and femininity. In 1973, for example, Yalom, Green, and Fisk, psychiatrists at Stanford University Medical Center, studied the effects of prenatal estrogens on development of behavioral characteristics in boys. They thought "female" hormones were disastrous to "normal male" psycho-sexual development. After measuring assertiveness, aggression, and athletic ability in the boys they investigated, they found these skills to be less developed due to the "female" hormones.[65]

Within the controversy about the contribution of nature and nurture to the origin of human behavior, such results, which were abundant, are to be regarded as strengthening the position of the "nature" adherents. They legitimized further biomedical investigations into prenatal hormone effects on human behavior. Some feminists, however, extended the role of prenatal hormones to explain the human behavioral repertoire, which also reinforced the "nature" position. In 1974, Eleanor Maccoby and Carol Jacklin published the well-known book, *The Psychology of Sex Differences,* which presented an evaluation of psychological studies of sex differences based on literature from January 1966 to the spring of 1973. They compared the results of hundreds of studies in eighty-four tables to "attempt to establish precisely what the differences are that need to be explained."[66]

While the explanatory chapters stressed psychological factors, the authors acknowledged that since sex was obviously a biological as well as a social characteristic, biology was also an important factor:

> If biological sex turns out to be linked with psychological functioning, the study of this linkage should help to deepen our understanding of a more basic matter: the way in which biological 'predispositions' interact with the impact of social experience to shape the psychological make up of a person. . . . Of course, it is very difficult to know whether a psychological sex difference has a biological origin, but since sex itself *is* a biological variable, there is hope that something can be discovered concerning the role that sex hormones and other genetically linked aspects of the body's functioning play in influencing an individual's reaction to his environment. It will be just as important to know what functions are *not* affected as to identify those that are.[67]

Maccoby and Jacklin thus considered the biology of sex not only in the sense of possessing genitals, but also with respect to hormones and genes. Scientifically correct, they stressed that they were neither geneticists nor biologists and therefore lacked the expertise for conducting an in-depth investigation of these factors. Moreover, their familiarity with feminist criticism inspired them to write that the literature they investigated was based on "observations that almost inevitably must be biased to some extent."[68] They felt the only solution was to make greater efforts to evaluate the degree of observer bias. They did this themselves: "We are both feminists (of different vintages, and one perhaps more militant than the other!), and although we have tried to be objective about the value laden topics discussed in this book, we know that we cannot have succeeded entirely. We doubt, in fact, that complete objectivity is possible for anyone engaged in such an enterprise whether male or female."[69]

Maccoby and Jacklin narrowed the long list of psychological sex differences down to a few major differences substantiated by biological research results. To this end, they summarized the data on sex differences in three types of findings: unfounded beliefs about sex differences, fairly well-established sex differences, and differences with ambiguous results. According to the fairly well-established differences, girls tended to have greater verbal ability than boys, boys excelled in visual-spatial ability and mathematical ability, and males were more aggressive than females.[70] They wrote: "Biological factors have been most clearly implicated in sex differences in aggression and visual-spatial ability."[71]

They argued that the male's greater biological aggression was supported by the similar ways that male primates expressed aggression, that this characteristic was cross-culturally universal, and that levels of aggression were responsive to sex hormones. Nevertheless, Maccoby and Jacklin also believed that aggressive behavior could be learned: "There is plentiful evidence that it *is* learned. We argue only that boys are more biologically prepared to learn it."[72] They also argued that the male predisposition toward aggression could probably be extended to some degree to other behavior, such as dominance, competitiveness, and activity level. According to Maccoby and Jacklin, dominance in most humans was called leadership. Though they found that leadership was determined by more than dominance and by factors not linked to biological traits (such as persuasion and charisma), they ascribed the human characteristic "leadership" as a biological predisposition to males. Previously, Money and Ehrhardt had included the characteristics dominance, competitiveness and activity within the realm of action of prenatal hormones. Maccoby and Jacklin supported and extended those findings to new behavioral categories. Besides the prenatal hormones, they perceived a link between their results and the suggestion by biologists that a gene was responsible for certain behavioral differences between women and men. Maccoby and Jacklin referred to the existence of a recessive sex-linked gene that contributed to superior spatial ability. They found little evidence of sex linkage for any of the genetic determiners of other specific abilities, such as mathematical or verbal ability.

Despite Maccoby and Jacklin's great caution in supporting a biological basis for different types of behavior, these feminists contributed to the biological construction of female and male behavior and reinforced the biological explanations for sex differences in behavior. In linking dominance, verbal and spatial abilities, immune diseases, migraine, and childhood learning disorders to prenatal hormones or genes, they paved the way for the research of the 1980s.[73] Geschwind, Galaburda, Benbow, Stanley, and many others suggested that hormones affected not only the hypothalamus but also the entire brain by differences in structuring the right and left sides of the brain in males and females.[74]

Research questions concerning active female sexual behavior, inspired by feminism and the search for real differences by the feminists Maccoby and Jacklin, strengthened the idea that individuals are to some extent predestined for "male" or "female" behavior by their prenatal hormones. Women who studied female sexual behavior contributed to a conceptual change of female nature, whereas Maccoby and Jacklin did not. We, however, have to consider that they published their book two years after the book of John Money and Anke Ehrhardt. Its success obliged Maccoby and Jacklin to subscribe to prenatal hormone effects on brain development and later masculine or feminine behavior. They had to pass the "obligatory point of passage" in order to be taken seriously, especially as feminists. For their scientific reputation it was more favorable to be criticized by feminists than to ignore the outcome of Money and Ehrhardt's work. Maccoby and Jacklin's work was of great value to psychology, and they substantially reduced the growing list of psychological sex differences. They surmised the existence of bias in biology as well as in psychology; nevertheless, they presumed biological sex differences to be real, which meant that women were likely to learn different things from men. They acknowledged social factors but separated them from a biological basis. This separation appeared especially problematic in biological investigations into prenatal hormone effects on human behavior later in life.

Environmental Factors and the Biological Construction of Behavior

During the 1970s, more types of behavior came to be thought of as affected by prenatal hormones, while the feminist "nurture" position simultaneously affected neuroendocrinological research into human behavior. How did this effect arise, and how did scientists deal with this idea?

In 1977, David Quadagno, Robert Briscoe, and Jill Quadagno from the University of Kansas published an article that critically examined research into prenatal hormone effects on the behavior of animals and humans and that argued that factors other than hormones underlay the recorded phenomena.[75] In the 1960s and 1970s, most results that provided knowledge about prenatal hormone effects came from tests on animals and humans born with anatomical abnormalities in their sexual organs. The authors believed this factor was considerably more important for the development of behavior than researchers supposed. In animals, this situation resulted from experimental hormone treatments. The human population, however, consisted of pseudohermaphrodites, whose ambiguous genitals were the consequence of a malfunction in their prenatal hormones. The studies regarded pseudohermaphrodites as experiments of nature. This factor had not been examined in animals, and had been underestimated in humans. Quadagno, Briscoe, and Quadagno suggested that the parents of both humans and animals with such abnormalities would have different expectations of such offspring than of their normal progeny and would consequently rear their affected children in a different manner. They argued that the outcome of this rearing was erroneously ascribed to prenatal hormone effects, while the ambiguous signals of the parents toward their daughters with masculinized genitalia was much more likely to be considered the cause of tomboyish or nonmaternal behavior of girls in studies like the one by Money and Ehrhardt. They argued that basing judgments of behavior on interviews with the children and the parents inspired doubt as to whether these behaviors were facts or merely perceptions of the parents concerning their children, which, in turn, seriously affected the self-image of the children in question. The authors believed that the real question was: "Why are they so perceived by themselves and others?" They suggested that the label "tomboy" that Money and Ehrhardt applied to the "masculinized" girls was justified for the girls and their families, and that this label "actually precedes the appearance of tomboy behavior (if it exists) or it may at least lead to biased perceptions of behavior."[76]

The authors also wondered about the effects of the surgical corrections and hormone therapy on the children's behavior. They suggested that hormone replacement therapy confers "high energy-expenditure levels" which may be unrelated to maleness or femaleness in the brain. In fact, they questioned the feasibility of investigating the effects of prenatal hormones on brain development and behavior in humans. Their arguments about human behavior were reinforced by the criticism of the same model used for investigating animals. They proposed alternative explanations based on postnatal factors for both humans and animals.

Later, Froukje Slijper, a Dutch child psychiatrist, investigated the effect of being ill on the behavioral development of "masculinized" girls. She concluded: "The hypothesis that behavior is masculinized by exposure to androgen hormones during early stages of development cannot be supported by this study. Psycho-social factors such as the child being sick, and parents' doubts about the sex of the child seem to have more influence on gender role behavior than does androgenic hormone action."[77]

How did scientists investigating prenatal hormone effects in animals and humans react to the serious criticism from Quadagno, Briscoe, and Quadagno? In the 1980s, social influences on behavioral development of animals became a subject of study. Celia Moore formulated a theory that combined nonbiological learning aspects of maternal behavior with biological effects of hormones on the development of rat behavior. She found that the maternal behavior of rats was affected by the hormonal condition of the pups and that both factors influenced the pups' future behavior.[78] Later, Moore investigated the development of sexual behavior in rats by observing the way that rat mothers raise their offspring and suggested that maternal behavior mediated the effects of prenatal androgens on the development of sexual behavior.[79] Of course, the research designs used in Celia Moore's studies of rat behavior were not suited for research on humans.

Anke Ehrhardt and Heino Meyer-Bahlburg, a psychiatrist who collaborated with Ehrhardt in several articles on prenatal hormone effects on human behavior, attempted to account for the possibility that parental expectation of tomboyish behavior affected girls born with "masculinized" genitalia. They ascertained that there was no obvious parental encouragement of masculine behavior in the hormone-exposed girls.[80] John Money seemed to digress from the prenatal hormone paradigm in work based on a longitudinal study of children born with ambiguous sexual organs. He concluded that the children's gender identity or gender role seldom failed to parallel the sex assigned at birth, even if genetic sex or genital anatomy differed from the sex of rearing. Nevertheless, he did not consider the development of gender identity or gender role to be purely psychosocial in nature but believed this process resulted from interaction between the biology of the body (including the brain) and the surrounding environment. According to Money, the product of these interactions was "programmed" in the brain.[81]

In March 1981, the optimism of scientists about unraveling the biological backgrounds of behavioral development was reflected in a special issue of *Science* devoted to "sexual dimorphism." Normally, each issue of *Science* consisted of several articles, not necessarily about the same subject. The articles in this issue summarized the factors surrounding sex differences with respect to ontogeny, phenotype, and hormone-sensitive actions. The subjects discussed in the articles started with genetic differences and covered cells, tissue, organs, and finally, systematic effects of gender. The effects of hormones on behavior were considered in the last two of the eight articles. These articles mentioned the problem of social factors that obscure the picture. The end of the introduction to the sexual dimorphism issue reads: "Despite shortcomings in clinical studies [into human behavior], it is now well recognized that sex differences are programmed from the beginning of ontogeny, are needed for reproduction, and have many consequences not directly related to fertility."[82]

In the 1980s, researchers studying hormone effects on human behavior tried to solve the methodological problem of abnormal genitals by investigating another population. The growing population of children of mothers who had taken hormone prescriptions during pregnancy (called DES daughters and sons) seemed ideal for this purpose. Their genitals were usually normal,[83] and they entered hospitals with fertility problems and an increased risk of cervical cancer, which meant that they needed regular medical checkups and were available for research.

DES daughters and sons were good research subjects for several reasons in addition to their normal genitalia. They were far more numerous than people born as intersex. In the United States, hormone therapy for pregnant women had been prescribed for several million risk pregnancies between 1940 and 1971. Of the various synthetic hormones used, most had been synthetic estrogens and progestagens.[84] Scientists hypothesized the effects of the different hormones on the behavior of the DES daughters and sons to be "androgenic" or "anti-androgenic" (meaning "masculinizing" or "anti-masculinizing," that is, "feminizing"), according to the dualist function of hormones in the organization theory about brain differentiation in females and males. As some hormones were difficult to categorize according to their function, an intermediate category was created: "weak androgens." Scientists defined the "androgyneity" of a hormone on the basis of its effects on what they perceived as male or female behavior.[85]

The availability of this vast group of children whose mothers had taken hormone treatments increased scientific optimism about separating bio-logical from environmental factors. Some scientists viewed the existence of these groups as a guarantee for obtaining an understanding of the effects of the different hormones on brain development and behavior. According to Melissa Hines: "Although prenatal hormone levels cannot account completely for sex differences in human behavior, recent method-ological innovations and the availability of potentially large human subject populations may make it possible to define relations between specific hormones and specific aspects of sexually dimorphic behavior . . . thus perhaps leading to elucidation of the neural underpinnings of sexually dimorphic behavior in humans as well as in other mammals."[86] The prospect of elucidating the relationship between specific hormones and types of behavior meant, however, that the methodological problem of the distinction between biological and social factors faded into the background. In the 1980s, many articles appeared on the effects of prenatal hormones on the behavior of both animals and humans. What happened to the methodology problem?

The findings of most studies of children whose mothers had received hormone treatments during pregnancy remained problematic in their methodology of separating social from biological factors. Control groups (persons that served as a basis for comparison with the subjects of the investigation to eliminate social variables) proved difficult to find. The behavioral results of the test subjects had to be compared with individuals from a group in which the following factors could be ruled out: parental influences, social class, economic and educational background, age, and medical history. While several control groups were used in some cases to eliminate the different social factors, the investigators were unable to draw totally unequivocal conclusions about prenatal hormonal effects on behavior for any of the groups. Apparently, this problem could not be solved by increasing the number of control groups. Researchers in the field argued that an *interactional model* was required for progress in understanding complex phenomena such as gender identity and other aspects of gender-related behavior. Anke Ehrhardt hoped a *biosocial perspective* would enhance the study.[87] The problem was not solved, however. Rather, it was allayed by new terms: interactional models or biosocial perspective.

In addition to the social factors, biological factors (the hormones) presented more complications than had been anticipated. Retrospective treatment data collected from physicians or hospital records were difficult to retrieve and were frequently imprecise with respect to timing, dosage, and even the type of hormone used in the treatments.[88] These data were very important, since "it depends on the type of drug and dosage whether the effect is androgenic or the opposite."[89] Ehrhardt also found that normal sexual organs turned out to be a mixed advantage. "This is an advantage in terms of a less confounding effect of the appearance of the sex organs at birth than in the high androgen syndromes (intersexes), it also means that it is entirely inferential whether the development of the fetus was indeed affected by the exogenously administered sex steroid or not."[90]

Notwithstanding the acknowledgment of the importance of social factors in the development of behavior in animals and humans and the difficulty of separating social factors from biological factors and of establishing biological variables, biomedical researchers persisted. As a result of these obstacles, however, researchers exercised greater caution in their conclusions about the effects of prenatal hormones on human behavior: Results were discussed in considerably greater detail during the 1980s and the length of these discussions increased accordingly.[91]

While some scientists have started to question the organization theory, most continue to adhere to it. Based on the immense number of results to this effect, they believe that prenatal hormones cause the brains and behavior of animals and humans to be "sexually dimorphic."[92] Nevertheless, this idea was also challenged in conceptual respects.

"Sexually Dimorphic" Behavior Challenged

In the 1970s, results were also published that conflicted with "sex dimorphism" in behavior. Which ideas formed the basis for this research? How successful was the attempted explanation that transcended the boundaries between sex dimorphism in brain development and behavior in humans?

Feminist views of the relationship between masculinity and femininity began to play a role in research on prenatal hormone effects in humans. Some feminists suggested that the traditional roles of both women and men could be replaced by androgynous role models. In these models, men and women could develop characteristics traditionally associated with the other sex; several such models were proposed. According to other feminists, however, androgyny is normative for women, and such models would prescribe that women integrate "masculine" aspects into their personality. In fact, they force women into a cultural ideal that contradicts the feminine. Moreover, they argued, these models implicitly accept the characteristics associated with femininity as socially inferior. For their part, supporters of the androgyny models argued that femininity did not exist independently and was merely the result of oppression. They found these models strategically important for avoiding biological determinism or essentialism.[93]

Once again, feminist thought concerning androgyny appeared to have the potential for introducing new behavioral categories into the realm of prenatal hormones, notwithstanding the fact that the consequences of the integration of these ideas impeded their scientific acceptance. Why did scientists have so much trouble accepting these results?

Publications by Sandra Bem and other feminist psychologists about changes in the concepts of masculinity and femininity in psychology affected research on the action of hormones on behavioral categories. In 1972, Bem published "The Measurement of Psychological Androgyny," in which she rejected the dualistic definitions of masculinity and femininity in psychological studies from an explicitly feminist perspective. In accordance with the discussion on androgyny, Bem argued that these characteristics should not be considered a dualism (the opposite extremes of a single continuum), but rather that individuals should be assessed in terms of both their "masculine assertive and instrumental dispositions [and] their feminine expressive and yielding natures."[94]

In 1974, the American psychobiologist Richard Whalen from the University of California at Irvine, an authority on fundamental research on hormones and behavior in rodents, published an article that introduced a model in which masculinity and femininity in behavior could develop independently of one another in the same individual.[95] Whalen read Bem's work,[96] and he chose the same name as Bem for the revised conceptualization of masculinity and femininity—"orthogonal"[97] (see fig. 3.1).

In 1976, June Reinisch at the Department of Developmental Psychology at Columbia University in New York introduced this model into research on prenatal hormone effects in humans.[98] She thought, however, that "perhaps masculinity and femininity exist on one dimension only when hormone influence or its absence is extant over the period of development 'natural' to the organism's ontogeny."[99] Although the reasons remained unclear, Reinisch was suggesting that the orthogonal model be reserved for unnatural situations.

In 1977, June Reinisch and William Karow published the results of investigations in which they had applied the model in *Archives of Sexual*

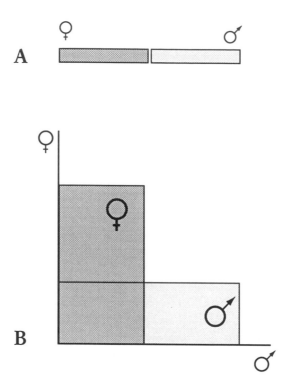

FIG. 3.1. Models of Femininity/Masculinity.

A. The dualistic model: Femininity is "not masculine," masculinity is "not feminine."

B. The orthogonal model, proposed in 1974: Femininity and masculinity are placed on different axes; they are characteristics that develop independently in an individual.

Behavior.[100] They compared three groups of persons whose mothers had been treated with progestins,[101] estrogens, or both types of hormones during pregnancy. They found the offspring of the progestin-treated mothers more independent, more individualistic, more self-assured, more self-sufficient, more sensitive, and less corteric than the offspring of the estrogen-treated mothers ("corteric" refers to "cortical alertness"—corteric individuals are more inclined to think than to feel). This group was reported to be more group-oriented, more group-dependent, more corteric, and less independent, less self-assured, and less sensitive. In the group with mothers that had been treated with both these hormones, they found an "intermediate" pattern of responses: They were more corteric, less independent, and less sensitive (like the estrogen group), and more self-sufficient (like the progestin-treated group). Reinisch and Karow noted that these differences did not correspond to a culturally stereotyped pattern of masculinization or feminization, but rather to a pattern of being "self" or "other" directed.

The gulf between the views of Reinisch and Karow and the traditional ideas of masculinity and femininity can be understood within the model they used, which in fact unified masculinity and femininity as human potentialities. As Reinisch stated in her 1976 article: "Hormone therapy appears to potentiate general dispositional tendencies which relate to the global organization of behavior."[102] Thus, according to Reinisch, hormones do not make brains male or female, but potentiate them toward human behavior in the broadest sense. While it is not certain whether Reinisch harbored this intention, she seems to have changed the ideas of the functions of hormones in the development of masculinity and femininity in the brain from *differentiating* between biological restrictions (called masculinity and femininity) to biologically *potentiating* different kinds of human behavior. This shift in the function of hormones can be seen as "prescribed" by the application of the orthogonal model in the experiments.

Remarkably, Reinisch published a paper in *Nature* based on these same investigations in 1977. For this article, she remodeled the data to reflect traditional beliefs about hormonal function in the development of masculinity and femininity in behavior. For the research reported in this article, she selected two smaller groups, treated either with estrogens or with progestins. Progestins were associated with the development of "self-directed" personalities, while estrogens were associated with "other-directed" personalities. Moreover, this article mentioned that the group treated with progestin achieved high scores on a test of personality factors identified as being closely related to school achievement and success. The group treated with estrogen scored poorly on this test. In this article, Reinisch described the progestin-treated group as "inner-" or "self-directed" and the estrogen treated group as "outer-" or "other-directed" but did not relate these labels to masculinity and femininity.[103]

Reinisch's application of the orthogonal model in her study of prenatal hormone effects in humans once again called attention to new characteristics within the prenatal hormone paradigm. This time, however, the characteristics ascribed to hormones were inclined to cross the boundaries of "dimorphism" in male and female behavior. How did scientists in the field react?

Melissa Hines, who published a dissertation on DES exposure and human sexual "dimorphic behavior,"[104] found the results published by Reinisch and Karow in *Archives of Sexual Behavior* "difficult to interpret";[105] they were incompatible with her conceptions of masculinity and femininity. Moreover, she criticized the methodology behind these results. Reinisch's model did not appeal to Hines or to other researchers in their investigations of the effects of hormones on human behavior. In fact, even Reinisch had already abandoned the model that broke away from dimorphisms in male and female behavior in her *Nature* article. Later, she published on the effects of hormones (synthetic progestins) with an "androgenic potential" and their relation to aggression in humans.[106] In this publication, "androgenic" hormones resume their one-on-one relationship to traditional masculinity, which is expressed here as aggression.[107]

To understand Reinisch's reasons for abandoning her model and pursuing this new line of research, we must consider the following circumstances. In the first place, scientists generally adhered to the differentiation paradigm, according to which gonadal hormones were either androgenic or anti-androgenic, thereby respectively stimulating behavior considered masculine or feminine. If hormones were posited to have a potentiating function in the development of human behavior (thus crossing the boundaries of traditional masculinity and femininity), the differentiation paradigm would no longer have any meaning. In fact, Reinisch's study as published in *Archives of Sexual Behavior* undermined the organization theory. It is likely that few of her colleagues were prepared to challenge the idea of duality in the function of hormones. Apparently, Reinisch was not in a position to do so alone and certainly not as a woman scientist with ambitions.

In general it is almost impossible for a woman scientist to produce unconventional results, especially if they cross boundaries constructed by thousands of publications of male colleagues. Many female scientists have ambiguous feelings about criticism from a feminist perspective, perhaps even more so than male scientists. It is common that criticism from a feminist perspective is welcomed with skepticism or even with anger, as we learned from Leonore Tiefer's experiences. Therefore, women scientists formulating criticism mostly choose to do this from a scientific viewpoint rather than from a feminist standpoint. Reliance on the latter would be detrimental to their arguments and cogency. Criticism from a feminist perspective is easily dismissed by labeling it "not objective and thus not scientific." As explained in the first chapter, feminist ideas are suspect in this field of research. Moreover, for women scientists, the quality of their work is more important than the fact that they are female. Therefore, a distinction between feminist scientists and women scientists is hard to make. Be that as it may, women scientists with career ambitions also have to be careful in their support for boundary-crossing results such as those of Reinisch. This might be a reason for Hines's comments on Reinisch's unconventional results. It was safe to adhere to feminist ideas openly if a scientist's reputation was as firmly established as Beach's. He could point to "imbalance due to male investigators and theorists." Beach was in a position to do this; as we saw, it even improved his position. The suspicion of feminist ideas in this field probably also explains why Richard Whalen, a student of Beach, did not refer to Bem's work, though she obviously inspired him. His work was successful; it made most scientists abandon dualism in masculinity and femininity; Whalen's work meant that these concepts could be proposed as existing independently, at least in theory. In research, however, this "independence" was not translated to hormonal functions. Androgens continued to be considered chemical messengers for masculinity, and estrogens retained their function as vectors of femininity.[108]

In addition, the methods of selection used by scientific journals may have contributed to the publication and consequently the study of specific differential effects of androgenic or anti-androgenic hormones on behavior in terms of masculinization or the lack thereof, rather than to research on potentiating (or "independent") hormone effects on human behavior. Why else would Reinisch have remodeled her results for their publication in *Nature*? Results confirming the influence of biological factors in sex-dimorphic "male" and "female" behavior in general were easily published. Ruth Bleier pointed to this fact and noted several methodological shortcomings[109] in articles on sex differences in the human brain that appeared in *Science*.[110] In the 1980s the publication policy of accepting articles confirming biological differences in the brains of women and men, rather than articles that did not, reflected a culturally dominant view of the sexes as "biologically dimorphic." Although in general difference is more interesting than equality in science, it is remarkable that articles with such methodological shortcomings are published in a journal with the high standards of *Science*.

The dominance of this view on the sexes, is also apparent, however, in the strategies used for popularizing this type of research. Journalists gave increasing publicity to the idea that prenatal hormones caused male or female brains and behavior, in spite of scientists' care for proper methodology and conclusions and even occasional doubts about the prenatal hormone paradigm.[111] In 1989, two journalists, Anne Moir and David Jessel, published *BrainSex: The REAL Difference between MEN and WOMEN*. They argued that the social explanation for sex differences in behavior was inadequate, and the assertion that men and women were equal in aptitude, skill, and behavior was tantamount to building a society based on a biological and scientific lie. Moir and Jessel proposed a "pacification between the sexes" and suggested that relationships would improve by accepting that women and men differ biologically. Feminists are portrayed as advocates of a denial of human nature, thus as frustrating women and men by urging women to compete for jobs and men to rear their children.[112]

According to Moir and Jessel, men's neural structuring gives them a congenital advantage in mathematics, physics, abstract thought, and all sports requiring hand-eye coordination. Compartmentalization of their brain and thus their various mental states makes it difficult for them to express emotions (right brain) verbally (left brain). Most comfortable in object relations and naturally aggressive, men are promiscuous, competitive, and less emotional than women. Women's linguistic acuity, sensory receptivity, and extensive interconnection between brain functions makes it easier for them to synthesize information ("women's intuition"). Women show an aptitude for all activities involving interpersonal relations (mothering, teaching, nursing). People-oriented, sensitive, and emotional, they are generally monogamous and sacrifice prestige and gain for social cohesion. Women are more interested in pretty clothes and a clean house, can do different things at the same time and are better equipped to cope with stress. Moir and Jessel attributed all these differences to hormones, although it is not a prenatal on-off event but a repeated process that generates the physically sexed body parts, the appropriate brain structure, and the mechanisms of sexual arousal. Any malfunction in these hormonal baptisms would make a child "abnormally" male or female.

What is the basis for Moir and Jessel's positive arguments? The references suggest an impressive basis of hundreds of scientific publications. Critical articles, however, are absent from their list—those by colleagues of the cited authors, for example, the one by the Quadagnos and Briscoe; publications by feminist biologists with fundamental criticisms, such as those by Ruth Bleier, Ruth Hubbard, and Lynda Birke, do not show in their references. Moir and Jessel do refer to the book by the feminist biologist Anne Fausto-Sterling, but negatively. They have her argue that publications on sex differences are a waste of paper, meant to maintain a scientific misunderstanding. Thus, they simply subject her work to ridicule. In their text they lead us to believe that all scientists investigating this subject subscribe to their ideas without the slightest doubt. They do not tell the reader about any difficulties scientists have in establishing a causal relationship between prenatal hormone effects and later behavior in DES children, or between the different brain structures and what it means for our behavior. The call for biosocial research models in order to investigate biological and social factors and their possible interactions on the development of behavior remains unheard. And they do not cite examples showing that there is a relationship between social factors and hormone levels in the blood of animals and humans. According to Moir and Jessel, beliefs, the different capacities of men and women are the result of, not surprisingly, "male" and "female" hormones.

Notwithstanding the (too) positive message and the doubtful scientific underpinnings, the book was successful. It was reviewed in many journals and newspapers in Europe and the United States. Some reviews were rather skeptical, but others suggested reconsidering female emancipation.[113] Journalists popularized the book in their turn and made the story even more juicy. The Dutch *Panorama*, for example, provided men with a biological basis for being more egoistic. And, of course, the argument was that we should all accept each other's biological inclinations. The result would be that men do not have to take seriously their spouses' desire for a career if they don't like the idea. Women, being less egoistic, will easily accept their partner's biological urge to be promiscuous; men, of course, cannot accept that in their wives—it would be doubly unnatural. It is, however, quite convenient that nature allows women to do more things at the same time and provides them with a more sophisticated biology to cope with stress; this is especially true in societies that demand both that women work and that they organize a household with children. To be a "real" woman and to be happy, a woman needs children. A man's nature, made to compete, will become frustrated if he takes care of his children, etc. Any stereotype about the sexes fits into Moir and Jessel's image of "nature."

Positing a biological background for differences between women and men is popular. We can compare the situation at the end of the century with that at its beginning, during the "first feminist wave." At that time the argument was that women's brains were smaller than those of men, therefore they lacked the intelligence to study and to vote. The male and female characteristics that Moir and Jessel ascribe to biological differences are in perfect keeping with our times. People recognize themselves and others; it all seems quite plausible. Arguments such as those of Moir and Jessel have a forceful cogency. One indication of the popularity of the idea of "biologically dimorphic" behavior in women and men is Moir and Jessel's success with an hours-long television series on sex and the brain. It has been shown in Canada, on the U.S. Discovery Channel, in the Netherlands, and most likely also in other European countries.

Conclusions

From 1959, the beginning of the research based on the organization theory, until the mid 1970s, researchers used circular reasoning to match androgens, male brains, and sexual and nonsexual activity in experiments as masculine. Although this research was methodologically objective, the results in behavioral neuroendocrinology were colored by the people asking the research questions and constructing the experimental designs.[114] The rise of the women's movement and the introduction of women researchers changed the questions asked, and new research designs were constructed that provided completely new research results concerning female sexual behavior. We may conclude that feminism affected behavioral neuroendocrinology in several areas. The status of female rodents in experiments changed; they were no longer a mere test medium for investigations of male development. Research on female development generated a need for new concepts in studying female behavior. Moreover, the theory on prenatal hormone effects on brain development was modified. After Beach's article appeared in 1976, females were seen as having a section in their brain that controlled their sexual behavior—an asset that had been reserved for males until then.

Feminist thought in general, and especially female novices in science, opened up the masculine circle and shed light on the feminine. In most cases this was done from a scientific rather than from a feminist perspective, and the work became "incorporated" into this field of science without calling the standards for scientific objectivity into question. Nevertheless, due to feminism, the dualism in the organization theory, or rather the monism of masculinity in the brain, which precluded the existence of "the feminine," was transformed into a dichotomy of masculinity and femininity. In Laqueur's terms, the one-sex model was replaced by a two-sex model. Like the controversy he described concerning the rise of the two-sex model during the Enlightenment, the body-mind or nature-culture opposition became problematic.[115]

Which conditions enabled feminist ideas to become integrated into science? In neuroendocrinology, the ideas of women researchers or feminists could become integrated as long as they contributed to the idea of a dichotomy between the sexes and subscribed to the prenatal hormone paradigm. These notions turned out to be the same, as the vicissitudes of Reinisch's research indicate. She subscribed to the prenatal hormone paradigm, but in a way that undermined the idea of the dichotomy between the sexes. Her theory about the function of hormones and human behavior originated in the idea of potentiating rather than differentiating behavior, as the organization theory prescribed. Apparently, the scientific community was not receptive to this approach in 1977.

Other conditions can also determine the possibilities for integrating scientific and feminist ideas, or rather, they affect the pace of integration. For example, the new insights into female sexual behavior proved very valuable in the competition to produce knowledge within and between disciplines. For Doty, and especially for Beach, publishing material about aspects of female sexual behavior presented opportunities for reconstituting the scientific reputation of psychology as the preeminent discipline in studies of behavior. This point of view is strengthened by considering the fact that Beach not only developed the new definitions of female sexual behavior but also acknowledged the validity of the organization theory for investigations into the development of sexual behavior in the same article. We may regard this act as a negotiation about knowledge concerning sexual behavior: Beach finally "offered to give up" his psychological model focusing on experience and learning for the model of organization by hormones of parts of the brain controlling sexual behavior. As a result, Beach was readmitted to the discussion between mainstream researchers in the field who subscribed to the organization theory. Moreover, he regained his authority in scientific respects on the effects of hormones in adult and prenatal life. Reputation as a factor in the mechanism of acceptance of new insights cannot be ignored. This factor also counted for Maccoby and Jacklin's work. They reduced the growing list of psychological sex differences to a few. If Maccoby and Jacklin had not suggested a biological basis for these differences, their work would have had little impact.

Another factor that favored the acceptance of the new insights in the scientific community was the introduction of a new domain in scientific research following Beach's article: female brain development and female sexual behavior, which could be studied as the result of prenatal hormone effects. Had Beach not based his new support for the organization theory on studies of female sexual behavior, female sexuality would probably not have been located in the brain as early as 1976. Until then, researchers had focused on the effects of hormone injections on sexual behavior in adult female animals. Moreover, universal acceptance of the new concepts for studying female behavioral categories would have proceeded far more slowly.

The conditions for integrating feminist ideas as described above are closely connected to another factor, which is probably the prerequisite for the former conditions. This aspect involves culturally (and thus scientifically) accepted views of "feminine" or "masculine" behavior. In the 1970s, women researchers provided new insights into active female sexual behavior, while feminism and the introduction of oral contraceptives promoted a growing cultural basis for extending the scope of femininity to include an active sexuality. Scientists had previously published objections concerning the neglect of active female sexual behavior in rats, thereby creating a cultural and scientific environment for research like the studies by Monica Schoelch-Krieger and others who followed in her footsteps.

By contrast, cultural support for Reinisch's research was virtually nil. Her 1977 publication in *Archives of Sexual Behavior* had additional implications for both femininity and masculinity; her results actually dissolved these categories. Even feminist views of the 1990s lack a consensus about this as opposed to attitudes about active female sexual behavior.

These arguments provide a basis for evaluating Longino's theoretical opinion that feminists stabilized the dichotomy between the sexes as much as they undermined it. The validity of this argument depends on the dichotomy concerned: the dichotomy in which "femininity" is absent, or the dichotomy in which "femininity" appears as the opposite of masculinity.

The proposal of the 1959 theory about brain development dates from an era when few women researchers were in a position to generate theories, ask research questions, or develop research designs *as women*. The few active women scientists usually just accepted scientific theories, research questions, and methods, which were considered the only theories, the only questions, and the only methods. While some exceptions are known, women who offered original insights, these insights tended to be credited to their male supervisors or colleagues.[116] Before and during the 1950s, women scientists were not perceived as women in the way that their male colleagues were viewed as men. It is thus hardly surprising that the 1959 proposal of the theory about differentiation of the brain also failed to include "the female." One of feminism's achievements is the opportunity for researchers to exist as women that has been available since the 1970s. Both the questions asked by these women and their results have extended the prenatal-hormone paradigm to include femininity and a further biological dichotomization of behavior. Furthermore, their reinforcement of the dichotomy actually undermined the monism in which femininity is a gaping void.

Female and male scientists, such as Bem, Reinisch, and Whalen, challenged the theoretical basis of the biological dichotomy. This act met with resistance from experimental circles, at least in behavioral neuroendocrinology, which was hardly cause for amazement in a period when dominant cultural thought about the sexes remained dichotomous, whether in biological or cultural respects (as most feminists believed), or as an interaction between the two forces (as most biologists believed).

Despite scientists' methodological care and cautious conclusions, cultural views consider the dichotomy between the sexes and other behavioral features a *biological* phenomenon. This outlook is most clear in the eagerness of journalists to popularize scientific results that consolidate the scope of biological femininity and masculinity. In general, however, researchers in various disciplines are manifesting a growing interest in biological factors (e.g., genes, serotonin) that affect human behavior.

These findings are thus in keeping with Helen Longino's argument that as long as dimorphisms called masculinity and femininity remain at the center of feminist discourse, other patterns of difference remain hidden, both as possibility and as reality. Longino argues that the etiology of gender, role behavior, and sexual orientation is too complex to be conveyed by describing it as sex-dimorphic. In particular, the idea remains submerged that a multiplicity of modes of personality organization is linked to sex and sexuality—a multiplicity of genders constructed at the intersection of biological sex, sexual orientation, reproductive status, class, race, and sexual ideology.[117]

4

THE CONSTRUCTION OF WOMEN AND
MEN IN MEDICAL PRACTICE

Introduction

In the preceding chapters we saw how the prenatal hormone theory became an "obligatory point of passage"[1] after the publication of Money and Ehrhardt's investigations into prenatal hormone effects on the behavioral development of pseudohermaphrodites.[2] That is to say, everyone involved in the development of gender identity or role was obliged to refer to it for the sake of cogency. In 1955, before the appearance of the organization theory, John Money and his colleagues, who worked with intersexes, saw masculinity or femininity in behavior as the result of experiences in growing up.[3] By 1972 they had modified that position: Male or female behavior became at least partly the result of prenatal hormone bathing of the brain. Especially in medical practice, the theory enhanced the insight into the development of their masculine or feminine behavior on the part of physicians and psychiatrists working with people born with ambiguous genitals. Treatment designed to help people born with ambiguous genitals become "real" women or men currently supplements hormones and surgery with psychological counseling.[4]

Even though most pseudohermaphrodites are not physically ill, doctors and psychiatrists consider the available methods of treatment extremely beneficial. In Western culture a life in which an individual's sex is a subject of ambiguity is virtually inconceivable.[5] Even our language reflects experiences within our sexualized society.[6] Doubts concerning the sex of a child are considered a medical rather than a social problem. In such cases, medical treatment serves to adapt a person's body to social environment. Stefan Hirschauer has demonstrated how surgery actually constructs the body to function as a bearer of cultural significances, with genital surgery being an outstanding example.[7]

This chapter deals with perceptions of "normal" men and women among professional health care workers treating pseudohermaphrodites. Moreover, I consider how images of masculinity and femininity in fundamental biomedical knowledge as revealed in the previous chapter are reflected in the treatment of individuals.[8]

During the period under consideration (1972–1989), ideas of "normal" femininity changed. Medical teams treating pseudohermaphrodites began to devote more attention to female sexuality. Nevertheless, the decision to attribute a female or male sex clearly indicated that in "making" a woman, present and future reproductive prospects carried more weight than sexual function.

This analysis highlights images of "normal" masculinity and femininity that reflect traditional views. To understand the manifestations of these traditional images in treatments of pseudohermaphrodites I have compared them with the images of femininity and masculinity in fundamental biomedical research. The images applied in the treatment of pseudohermaphroditism appear to conflict with the views used in biomedical research. While fundamental researchers could afford to produce carefully balanced knowledge, professionals treating pseudohermaphrodites preferred to use unambiguous criteria as a basis for their decisions. Given the high degree of task-uncertainty that has always characterized medical practice, mechanisms to reduce this insecurity were desirable.[9] The simplification of results in fundamental research exemplifies this ambition.[10] First, let us examine perceptions of intersexuality in times and places lacking the scientific understanding and medical treatments.

Pseudohermaphroditism through the Ages

Intersex children have entered our world in times and places where the urge and knowledge to provide people with a distinct sex did not exist. In antiquity, the union of male and female bodily characteristics in an individual was a favorite motif. Such individuals can even be found among the gods. Hermaphroditus, the son of the god Hermes and the goddess Aphrodite, was an androgynous deity. This motif also figured in matriarchal religions.[11] Some societies not yet ruled by the tenets of Western science accept pseudohermaphrodites as a third sex. In New Guinea, for example, researchers have discovered a culturally integrated third sex.[12]

Suzanne Kessler and Wendy McKenna list more examples in *Gender: An Ethnomethodological Approach*.[13] They describe people in American Indian societies called berdaches, who were usually males lived their lives as females, although there were also instances of females who lived their lives as males. People similar to berdaches have also been found in Alaska, Siberia, Central and South Asia, Oceania, Australia, Sudan, and the Amazon region. Although it is unclear whether all these people are actually pseudohermaphrodites, other cultures seem to afford more opportunities for adopting another gender and sometimes even acknowledge this condition separately from the male/female framework.

The berdaches are regarded with great esteem. The status of their counterparts in other societies is considerably lower, although they are generally tolerated. Kessler and McKenna note the difficulty encountered by Western observers in understanding these phenomena, since they look for signs that fit their own gender criteria. This problem is apparent in reports of berdaches written earlier in this century, before anthropologists questioned the universality of their organizing concepts with regard to gender.

European historiography has always viewed the existence of a third sex as an impossibility. Most cases of children that did not clearly belong to either sex were discovered and classified by physicians as pseudo-hermaphrodites.[14] In eras when they lacked the knowledge and the skills to adapt such children to a specific sex, physicians conferred in deciding about their fate. Often, their task involved advising judicial officials, and sometimes the clergy also became involved. Over time, physicians and officials adjusted their approach to people born as intersex according to the prevailing explanation of their existence in relation to "normal" mankind. Julia Epstein described the growing interest in natural history in the sixteenth century that led to a shift in the treatment of pseudo-hermaphrodites: From being sacrificed as monsters, considered to be nonhuman threats to humanity, they became "naturally anomalous."[15] According to Randolph Trumbach, in Western societies, fear of punishment for being homosexual made it especially difficult for pseudo-hermaphrodites.[16] In this period, physicians assumed their responsibility for preventing humans from crossing the gender boundaries imposed by law and morality. Pseudohermaphrodites were jailed or had every sexual organ surgically removed to prevent sexual feelings.

Eighteenth-century scientists began to advocate an understanding of the relationship between the anomalous and the normal, which resulted in commentaries on the role of the male and female seed in reproduction as dictated by the science of "generation." In the nineteenth century, early embryology developed the germ layer theory, which substituted this explanation for the phenomenon. In this theory, the sexual organs of the male and female share common origins. These scientific explanations, however, did not bring about social acceptance of pseudohermaph-rodites.[17]

The twentieth century offered yet another explanation: Scientists ascribed anomalous genitals to abnormal hormone levels before birth. Until the 1940s, however, no scientifically based treatment for pseudo-hermaphrodites was available except surgical removal of their gender-crossing genitals. This situation changed during the 1950s. Alfred Jost from the Collège de France submitted a theory about the effects of hormones on the development of genital organs prior to birth. According to his theory, an individual develops external male genitals when androgens are present in the blood of the fetus; when no androgens are present, the fetus develops female genitals.[18] Since the 1950s, scientists have regarded development of the male as a modification of female development: Male genitalia are created by the addition of "something masculine" (i.e., androgens).[19] Pseudohermaphrodites' deviant genitalia are thought to be the result of an abnormal hormonal situation during the prenatal period. Jost's theory provided experimental scientific insight into the existence of pseudohermaphrodites and led to an extension of medical treatment. Henceforward, physicians could prescribe hormones to people born as intersex.

As explained in the previous chapter, since the publication of the work of John Money and Anke Ehrhardt on the effects of prenatal hormones on the behavioral development of pseudohermaphrodites, physicians and psychiatrists have assumed prenatal hormone imbalances affected male or female development of the brain. This process would cause pseudoher-maphrodites to differ psychologically from "normal" men and women.[20] Authors who published on treatment of pseudohermaphrodites therefore advocated better psychological counseling. Their motivation was not only the general belief among physicians that psychological guidance was important for accomplishing their work; it also emerged from their concern regarding the consequences of abnormal effects of hormones on pseudohermaphrodites' brain development into masculine or feminine, as the following passage illustrates: "[Results] suggest that a direct effect of androgen on the developing fetal brain is at least a complementary, and perhaps a more important, explanation of the . . . findings. . . . It is likely that accompanying psychological support, based on an improved understanding of the patient's psychosexual status could also help."[21] Based on this knowledge, doctors strongly recommended providing pseudoher-maphrodites with the best possible assistance for becoming female or male in psychological respects as well. The emergence of knowledge about prenatal development of genitals and brains enhanced doctors' scientific understanding and certainty in diagnosing and treating children with ambiguous genitals. Although the decision about treatment is frequently difficult, medical possibilities for adapting people to either sex are almost exhaustive in external respects. Most surgery is, however, cosmetic and scarring leads to loss of orgasm in many cases.[22]

Medical Considerations in the Treatment of Ambiguous Sex

When do physicians apply the designation "pseudohermaphrodite" in children? In most cases of pseudohermaphroditism, a deviation of the genital organs can be observed at birth. The baby's clitoris may be shaped like a penis, or the penis may be so small that it resembles a clitoris. Sometimes, the labia or testes of these children are not properly developed either. Scientists have distinguished several causes that can lead to the hormonal imbalance before birth to which they ascribe the development of ambiguous genitals. In genetic females (XX chromosomes), the adrenal gland can produce abnormal amounts of hormones, which result in masculinized genitals. This form of pseudohermaphroditism became well known through the studies of Money and Ehrhardt, who designated such individuals as CAH girls or "tomboys." In some cases, hormone medication of the mother during pregnancy to prevent miscarriage (DES) led to the birth of a girl with masculinized genitals.

In genetic males (XY chromosomes), an enzyme deficiency can disturb the production of androgens necessary for the development of the male sexual organs, resulting in a small penis or a sort of vagina. Alternatively, a complete or partial insensitivity to androgens results in the development of a female sexual organ: The baby is born as a girl without any interior sexual organs and is therefore sterile. Depending on the cause, the estimated incidence of such cases is 1 out of every 5,000 to 64,000 births.[23] Although the incidence of each individual abnormality is fairly low, the frequency of all forms of pseudo-hermaphroditism together make the chance of meeting a person with some form of pseudohermaphroditism not as rare as is commonly believed. Fausto-Sterling scoured the medical literature for frequency estimates and ended with a figure of 1.7 percent of all births. At the rate of 1.7 percent, this means that a town like Amsterdam, with 800,000 inhabitants, would have 13,600 people with varying degrees of intersexual development.[24] This number is still based on an estimate; but even if the occurrence were overestimated by a factor of two, Amsterdam would number 6,800 pseudohermaphroditic persons among its inhabitants. We do not see them or hear about pseudohermaphroditsm very often because we are dressed and as we can imagine, these persons or their parents keep silent. Moreover, pseudohermaphroditic babies may appear outwardly normal at birth, and abnormal development of the genitalia may occur later in life, sometimes as late as or even after puberty. A girl may not start menstruation, or a boy may not develop a beard. Sometimes, doctors consider such features a form of pseudohermaphroditism. In those cases, and also in non-pseudohermaphrodites, they relate the function of hormones to other bodily characteristics, the "secondary" sex characteristics. In cases labeled pseudohermaphroditism, physicians described bodily characteristics considered deviant from normal female or male, even if they did not judge them serious enough to warrant treatment. In the descriptions, normal physical appearances of women and men differ in development of breasts, muscles, distribution of body fat, body hair, height, and voice. Physicians have prescribed hormone therapy to help women develop breasts that conform more closely to normal appearance. Sometimes they also hope for an additional effect on the hair growth of such women. To help men with breasts acquire a normal masculine figure, they have often advised surgical correction.[25]

According to a description of an intersex woman, a muscular and tall physique does not reflect the normal appearance of a woman; normal is a "female" distribution of body fat,[26] no hair on the face or legs, and a "female" distribution of pubic hair. For men, the descriptions mention only beard growth. Also, a deviance of "secondary" sex characteristics may elicit a request for medical help, which can sometimes lead to the diagnosis of pseudo-hermaphroditism: Such complaints may range from problems with menstruation, to excessive hair growth or development of breasts, to deviant genital organs.

Nowadays, interdisciplinary teams are responsible for diagnosis of and therapy for pseudohermaphrodites. These teams recommend intervention as soon as possible after the birth of a pseudohermaphroditic baby since most parents find it difficult to accept a child with an ambiguous sex.[27]

Which criteria affect the medical decision to "make" such children into girls or boys? Genetic sex appears to be an important criterion. For women, it is decisive: Doctors usually "make" a girl when a child has two X chromosomes. When the child is a boy in genetic respects (XY chromosomes), however, the size of the penis is decisive. If the penis of an

XY-boy is of a certain minimum size, the team decides to help the child become a boy. If not, a vagina is created, and the child is "made" into a girl.[28]

Doctors involved in the treatment of a girl often mention the depth of her vagina, which ends blindly in some cases. When such girls reach adulthood, physicians advise these women to keep their vaginas "at depth" by engaging in regular sexual intercourse or with plastic devices. Apparently, treatment of pseudohermaphrodites is closely related to ideas regarding the functioning of the penis or vagina in heterosexual intercourse.[29]

The teams involved in treating pseudohermaphrodites, like many others, define sexual intercourse according to the functions of sexuality and reproduction, and therapy for both sexes reflects this distribution. They consider the ability of pseudohermaphrodites to engender children indicative of the success of the treatment. Upon closer examination, the treatment of women and men reflects different emphases with regard to sexual pleasure. The following motivation for the decision to alter the sex of a four-year-old boy indicates the different valuations of the importance of sexuality and fertility with respect to women and men: "We recommended a change to the female sex mainly because the penis was so tiny that a normal sexual life in the male role seemed most unlikely whereas fertile life in the female sex was clearly possible."[30]

The doctors in the preceding example explicitly weighed male sexuality against female fertility. "Normal" male sexuality was perceived in terms of heterosexual intercourse, which they did not consider feasible for this child. It is striking that the writers did not refer to the sexual options of the child as a woman, whereas they did mention the possibility of fertility as a woman.

The following passage also stresses the importance of intercourse for successful manhood: "Secondary male-sex characteristics began to appear at the age of 12 years and developed normally. He shaved daily and had sexual intercourse with ejaculation twice weekly."[31] Maybe this team considered male and female contributions to reproduction equally important, but they did not distinguish the male reproductive role from the ability to ejaculate. While the ability of healthy men to engender offspring does indeed correspond to the ability to ejaculate, the articles in question did not reveal whether this successful male pseudohermaphrodite was also capable of procreation.

Many articles from the beginning of the 1970s onward showed that female sexuality was of secondary importance in treating pseudoher-maphroditism. At that time, the problem of a deviant clitoris (usually too large) was normally solved by complete surgical removal of the organ: "After careful consideration we decided to ease the fulfillment of her female role by surgical and hormonal therapy. A clitoris extirpation and vaginal plastic surgery were performed."[32] Most doctors (and probably the women concerned as well) apparently considered the ability to have sexual intercourse desirable, even though the patients were infertile. Were these doctors not aware that the clitoris is essential for female orgasm? Or did they consider a woman's sexuality less important than her fertility and female role?

Nowadays, reduction of an enlarged clitoris is considered preferable to amputation. Remarkably, no public discussion about the advantages of reduction over amputation appears in the journals analyzed, or in the medical textbooks consulted on this subject.[33] Overall, the anatomical possibility for heterosexual intercourse appears to be an important indicator of normal manliness, whereas fertility serves as the most important criterion for normal womanliness. The next section will also show how this impression emerged from psychological counseling received by pseudohermaphrodites.

Treatment of Psychological Masculinity and Femininity

According to Money and Ehrhardt's hypothesis, the abnormal hormone levels underlying the deviant genital organs of pseudohermaphrodites also affect the development of their brains. Money and Ehrhardt considered pseudohermaphrodites to be experiments of nature, comparable to biological experiments with animals in laboratories. In 1972, a book appeared about their research that described the influence of androgens before birth on "sex-dimorphous" behavior such as the amount of energy expended in sport and games, the preference for certain ways of dressing, ambitions with regard to a career or motherhood.[34] Sexual tendencies (heterosexual, homosexual, or bisexual) were also causally connected with prenatal androgen levels.[35] In the book they published in 1972, Money and Ehrhardt suggested a relationship between the presence of androgens and a superior level of intelligence (IQ), an idea they discarded in subsequent works.

As the previous chapter described, Money and Ehrhardt's investigations sparked fierce criticism of the methodology used in their investigations into prenatal hormone effects on later behavior of pseudohermaphrodites. These remarks led Money and Ehrhardt to qualify their interpretations of the prenatal effects of hormones on later behavior in their more recent work. In 1980, Money no longer presented the effects of androgens before birth as direct causes of femininity and masculinity, but as tendencies toward masculine or feminine development.[36] Nevertheless, since the appearance of Money and Ehrhardt's book, many doctors (as well as laymen) have regarded sexual differences in behavior as largely affected by prenatal hormones. Doctors evaluating the results of surgery on pseudohermaphrodites ask not only whether sexual or reproductive capacities have developed, but also whether the behavior of those concerned has become distinctly masculine or feminine.

Like Money and Ehrhardt, physicians and psychiatrists treating pseudohermaphrodites view a sexual orientation toward women as a token of masculinity. Additional signs include aggressive, assertive, and energetic tendencies.[37] Working outside the home is also part of "normal" masculinity in the following quote: "In a domestic setting, the women take care of the household activities, while the affected subjects work as farmers, miners or woodsmen, as do the normal males in the town. They enjoy their role as head of the household."[38]

Femininity in behavior is regarded as being sexually oriented toward men and as showing ambitions for motherhood even if a woman is infertile: "Studies of psychosexual function suggest that these patients are feminine in behavior and outlook and function as normal adoptive mothers."[39] From another passage in a relatively recent publication, it emerges that doctors regard "tomboy"[40] behavior in girls as deviant feminine behavior, while their treatment was considered successful if a girl's interest shifted toward becoming physically attractive: "The staff were soon able to interest the child in female things, and she seemed particularly pleased by having ribbons of different shades in her hair each day . . . and the child became obviously feminine."[41]

Why do the images of masculinity and femininity applied in the treatment of pseudohermaphrodites appear so traditional? There are plenty of broad explanations (doctors are generally male, doctors generally have a conservative outlook, etc.). In my search for a more specific explanation, I focused on two aspects of the aid offered to pseudohermaphrodites: the fundamental knowledge on which treatment is based and the problems that characterize the assistance offered to pseudohermaphrodites.

Asymmetrical Duality within the Theory

The previous chapters showed that scientists conceptualized masculinity and femininity as a dualism in their experiments based on the theory about sexual differentiation in the brain. Masculinity equals the presence of androgens, whereas femininity equals their absence. In the description of pseudohermaphrodites, androgens are also seen as the cause of masculinity. Male activity involves primarily the active initiation of sex. The theory connects the absence of androgens with femininity. "Absence" and "femininity" also coincide in the description of pseudohermaphrodites. The absence of androgens corresponds to an absence of active sexuality. A woman is receptive, that is to say, receptive to male sexuality and capable of producing offspring. Thus, both in the 1959 theory on the male and female differentiation of the brain and in the treatment of pseudohermaphrodites, femininity and masculinity appear as an asymmetric duality.

It is significant, however, that the images of femininity and masculinity used by doctors in the 1970s and 1980s in the treatment of pseudohermaphrodites do not agree with the ideas addressed in biomedical research of that period. As we saw in the previous chapter, biomedical scientists in the 1970s began to focus on active female sexual behavior and moved away from asymmetrical dualities regarding masculinity and femininity. Moreover, partly due to the criticism of feminist researchers, the limitations of dualistic notions as such began to be recognized. Scholars proposed conceptualizing femininity and masculinity as independent of one another. The dualistic model used up to that time defined femininity and masculinity in terms that described both concepts: Feminine was not masculine and vice versa. In 1974, the psychobiologist Whalen presented a model that placed masculinity and femininity on different axes: They were independent from each other and indicated the behavioral capacities that might be available to an animal or human being[42] (see fig. 3.1).

Treatment of pseudohermaphrodites reflects few of these changes in basic science. Clearly, barriers exist between basic science and clinical medicine, and the application of fundamental knowledge in medical practice is a gradual process. Also, the application of such knowledge is subject to limitations and to doctors' views of usefulness. We have tried to understand how the transfer of basic knowledge about prenatal hormone effects on human development for use in medical practice led to the perpetuation of dualistic images of masculinity and femininity in the treatment of pseudohermaphrodites.

Transfer of Fundamental Knowledge into Medical Practice

Generally, when knowledge is transferred from fields where it was developed to be used in other fields, various subtle details are sacrificed.[43] Researchers in one field of study expect unequivocal answers from researchers in another field. Users of knowledge, such as doctors, are, if possible, even more interested in unambiguous information. I have identified three points relevant to the loss of such detail in treatment of pseudohermaphrodites.

In articles on the subject, doctors attribute many of their patients' symptoms to the absence or presence of androgens. A number of articles simultaneously address the effects of androgens before birth on the development of genital organs, the tendency to develop breasts, the development of the brain, and psychosexual orientation. In some cases, they even neglect to differentiate between statements about the short-lived, immediate effects of androgens on adults (such as their influence on the libido) on the one hand, and the supposedly permanent influence of hormones before birth on the other hand.[44] Their presentation of the effects of androgens on the development of genital organs, sexual identity, and sex-specific social roles as inextricably linked is equally striking. The descriptions of treatment for pseudohermaphrodites appear to equate masculinity with the activity of androgens. This tendency is even more remarkable, since the researchers oriented toward more fundamental types of research consider estrogen important in the development of the brain in both women and men. Case descriptions contain only occasional references to this function of estrogen, and the most recent medical textbooks do not mention the role of estrogens in the development of the brain, either. A recent textbook on endocrinology describes the function of hormones as follows: "The effects of testosterone are tissue specific and reflect the sum of the action as well as those of its conversion products."[45] The androgen "testosterone" is supposed to realize the differentiation of the brain, though part of the testosterone has to be converted first. Comparing this passage to current ideas in fundamental research on this subject shows that the sentence simplifies the concept tremendously.

The work of Money and Ehrhardt has also undergone simplification with use. Though Money and Ehrhardt eventually adopted a much more

balanced position concerning the effects of hormones on the differentiation of the brain and behavior in later publications than they had in 1972,
most passages cited in the work of the doctors studied refer to the book
published in 1972 or to even earlier works. This practice suggests that
Money and Ehrhardt's later work is too balanced and therefore too
ambiguous to serve as a guideline for the treatment of pseudohermaphrodites. Doctors need unambiguous knowledge. This need is one of
the reasons underlying the tenacity of traditional images of femininity and
masculinity in the articles concerning the treatment of pseudohermaphrodites.[46]

The doctor's need for unambiguous knowledge has its basis in medical
practice. Medical practice in general, and especially the area responsible
for the treatment of pseudohermaphrodites, involves a high degree of
task-uncertainty.[47] Differences of opinion about diagnosis and therapy, as
well as about steps to be taken by doctors, are commonplace. At the same
time, most patients (or their parents) want definitive answers. Doctors are
interested in providing such answers since they want to maintain their
patients' trust. Their patients' symptoms and problems are, in themselves,
causes of great uncertainty. Particularly among patients with ambiguous
genitals, unambiguous knowledge is more than welcome. Unequivocal
images of "normal" femininity and masculinity as therapeutic objectives
provide equal security. Moreover, doctors treat these people for uncertainty about their sex or gender. Living with such uncertainty is far from
easy in our society. Consequently, the desire for the greatest possible
clarity concerning sex may lead practitioners to invoke traditional norms
of masculinity and femininity.[48] In turn, treatment of pseudohermaphroditism revalidates old norms about "real" men and women.

Conclusions

Analysis of the medical construction of one sex or the other from
individuals of ambiguous sex reveals that variety in the sexes extends
beyond male and female, even in biological respects. This variety has
always been problematic in Western societies. In the twentieth century,
however, medical practice found solutions to the growing urge to "make"
two distinct sexes in anatomy as well as in behavior. In the 1950s,
biological theories about the development of genital organs created the
possibility for treating pseudohermaphroditism. At first, only anatomical
features were treated. Surgery was performed on ambiguous genital

organs and "secondary" sexual characteristics, such as breasts. Hormone treatments helped develop these organs or stimulate patterns of hair growth that were socially desirable for either sex. Later on, behavior was also assigned a biological sex by means of the theory of brain development. The work of Money and Ehrhardt served professionals treating pseudohermaphrodites in their psychological counseling of male or female patients.

Money and Ehrhardt, however, qualified their allegations, and medical practice required unequivocal criteria for decisions about the treatment of pseudohermaphroditism to reduce uncertainty. In this way, psychological treatment for pseudohermaphroditism contributed to a belief in perfect "sexual dimorphism" in the behavior of women and men.

In this context, it is understandable that simplifications in the study and treatment of human behavior do not have an arbitrary effect. Rather, they reflect the dominant cultural images of femininity and masculinity. So far, these images have made little allowance for the possibility of "normal" lesbianism or homosexuality. Many scientists and doctors are still looking for biological explanations for behavior that deviates from the "normal" male or female pattern, despite the balanced and even "cautionary" statements by biomedical scientists.[49] Within this context, sexually ambiguous bodies are shaped to form a heterosexual unity in both anatomical and psychological respects according to guidelines that emphasize sexuality in men and reproductivity and motherhood in women.

In spite of the system of values described above, some people born as pseudohermaphrodites in our society are grateful for the availability of medical knowledge that can make them either women or men. However, the numbers of intersex people who are not grateful are increasing. In England at least three support groups exist for women who have been born as intersex and in the United States a nascent movement to establish an intersex identity has appeared. Among the members are adults treated as children; from them we know that early genital surgery caused extensive scarring and led to loss of orgasm.[50] Even now, the possibility for medically treated intersex women to enjoy sexual pleasure is rarely mentioned, and serious follow up studies do not exist.

In evaluating such treatments I would question if a cultural context that makes it hard to exist without clearly belonging to one sex or the other is more important than taking the risk of multiple surgeries and thereby removing the possibility for sexual pleasure. This question should be raised for parents who ask medical help for a baby born as intersex as well as for adults diagnosed as suffering from some form of pseudohermaphroditism.

Images of femininity and masculinity have changed over the past few decades. Further examination of the images used in the treatment of pseudohermaphrodites is currently in order, and such trends can be observed. A recent publication has suggested that the image of male sexuality is changing. According to the authors, men with a micropenis appear to be able to enjoy sexual experiences.[51] It would be an immense step forward in science and medical practice if we could become aware of the contents of our dualist images of sex, sexuality, and gender; if those with responsibilities for producing knowledge and support for people's well-being could accept human diversity as it always exists instead of constructing nature according to such dual cultural images. I hope to live to see multiplicity of gender cherished at the intersection of biological sex, class, and race.

5

REINVENTING THE SEXES

In the previous chapter we saw gender teams constructing intersex people and helping them to meet the cultural need to be either male or female. This "construction" also implied behavior according to existing assumptions concerning "natural" masculinity and femininity. In this way medical practice takes care to maintain the duality of the sexes in terms of body, sexuality, and behavior—more or less according to the images of the sexes as constructed in laboratory research. We observed this construction in chapters 2 and 3. In chapter 3 we saw how scientists and feminists collaborated in bringing a growing number of human qualities into the realm of the prenatal hormone paradigm, although many feminists disputed biological claims about masculinity and femininity in behavior because the results confirmed traditional ideas about the sexes. In the case of the nondualistic model, the model in which masculinity and femininity could exist in one person, however, the behavioral results of the experiments no longer fit these traditional images. Chapter 2 related how dual images of masculinity and femininity were conditions for the scientific acceptance of the prenatal hormone paradigm: Presence of androgens, "male" hormones, made a brain masculine, absence of this chemical made a brain feminine. The similarity with Freud's thinking is striking: presence or absence of a penis is constitutive for being a man or a woman.

Chapters 2 and 3 demonstrated how scientists struggled with their questions for research, their methods, and their interpretations of results to fit their claims to culturally dominant images of masculinity and femininity. The struggle of scientists concerned "unruly" hormones, sexual behavior of females that had been overlooked previously, and the distinction between the effects of nature and nurture in their experiments. Finally, their claims formed a traditional argument in a period of debate about masculinity and femininity as well as the contribution of nature or nurture to these phenomena. In the previous chapter we saw that neither hormones nor behaviors and not even bodies turned out to fit permanently into the existing masculine-feminine dualism.

In this study the boundaries between masculinity and femininity as well as between nature and nurture are at issue. In scientific circles, especially since the 1970s, many assumed a link between genetic explanations for biological dispositions of male or female behavior, as theorized by sociobiologists,[1] and results based on studies of prenatal hormone effects. They believed that male or female genes (XY or XX) expressed themselves through hormones before birth. The success of research based on the organization theory was paralleled in other fields of research on biological backgrounds of behavior; this type of research expanded enormously, and many new scientific journals were founded in this area.[2] The optimism of scientists working in behavioral neuroendocrinology regarding the separation of the nature component from nurture influences was also reflected in other biomedical research into biological backgrounds of human characteristics that varied from behavior to predispositions for diseases. We can see the scientific desire to chart the human genome in the 1990s as an optimistic scientific prolongation of this type of research. As the nurture-nature debate is relevant to all these disciplines, I will relate it to the perspectives from the previous chapters.

First I want to return to the book's central question concerning scientists' and physicians' use of knowledge and practices originating from the organization theory in constructing dualist images of femininity and masculinity. I will also discuss the contribution of feminism to stabilization and change in these images.

To answer these questions, I will divide this analysis into three chronological periods. The first period (1959–1971) is characterized by unhindered progress in the research. Scientists investigated the effects of prenatal hormones on male brain development and behavior. They did not consider female brain development or cultural factors in behavioral development. In Laqueur's terms, we could say that the organization theory was a one-sex model.[3] During the second period (1971–1976), growing criticism emerged about issues such as the neglect of female aspects. Eventually, these objections led to the incorporation of the second sex in the prenatal hormone paradigm. The resulting two-sex model sparked questions about the effects of cultural factors on the development of behavior. Research conducted during the third period (1976–1985) focused on human brain development and behavior. Scientists were haunted by methodological problems associated with distinguishing the biological and cultural variables affecting the results they measured. For each period, I will begin by identifying the groups that became involved in the networks that accepted knowledge about the development of behavior and explanations for the phenomena observed.

I will present a chronology of the social and cognitive conditions that affected the interactions between these groups and the manner in which they changed images of masculinity and femininity.

Finally, I will introduce a model that eliminates any ontological difference between nature and nurture factors affecting behavior. This approach is justified, since the previous chapters have revealed that nature as such does not exist in laboratories. All what is investigated about nature is as cultural as knowledge about nurture effects on behavior. Of course this vision has implications for the sex-gender divide in feminist theory. I propose to maintain the distinction, but to abandon the separation. First I will take the reader back to 1959.

1959–1971: Masculine Monism

In this period, the production of knowledge based on the organization theory encountered no obstacles and was accepted with relative ease by the scientific community. The 1959 proposal of the organization theory by Charles Phoenix, Robert Goy, Arnold Gerall, and William Young ushered in the heyday of knowledge concerning the effects of prenatal hormones on future behavior among laboratory rodents. The prenatal hormone paradigm appealed to scientists in behavioral neuroendocrinology as well as to their counterparts in related biomedical disciplines such as embryology and endocrinology. Most scientists in these disciplines easily made the transition from considering the effects of androgens on male physiology to considering their effects on male sexual behavior.[4] Soon after the 1959 proposal, scientists studied prenatal hormone effects on all sorts of behavior in many animal species, including primates.

From the outset, the scientists who proposed the organization theory based on animal investigations proclaimed the importance of the theory for understanding human behavior. The theory also appealed to neurologists, psychiatrists, and many psychologists: The prenatal hormone paradigm promised a scientific answer to the old question concerning the biological origin of male homosexuality, considered to be a female sexual orientation.

In this period, other scientists specializing in the development of behavior were very receptive to neuroendocrinologists' knowledge. The most important condition for this acceptance was cognitive: The theory was based on ideas about the function of androgens as chemical messengers of masculinity and was compatible with knowledge accepted by all scientists involved in this network. Moreover, scientists in several fields soon shared this theory because its proposal created a need for a theory about the effects of prenatal hormones on the development of behavior.

Another favorable condition, social in origin, was that most scientists involved in the research in the 1960s were male and shared an interest in the development of male heterosexual and homosexual behavior.

In this period, scientists who accepted knowledge based on the prenatal hormone paradigm subjected images of femininity and masculinity to a radical reconstruction. Before 1959, scientists considered the prenatal brain asexual or bisexual. Feminine and masculine sexual behavior were thought to be *temporarily* affected by chemicals: Estrogens and androgens supposedly had an effect on sexual behavior during adult life only. The primary functions ascribed to estrogens by biomedical scientists involved female reproductive physiology, while those attributed to androgens concerned male reproductive physiology and sexuality. Scientists viewed the effects of these hormones as diametric opposites in that they were thought to have the reverse effect when applied to the "opposite" sex.

After 1959, theories about the effects of androgens (but not those concerning estrogens) were extended to prenatal life. Scientists accepted the proposition that androgens *permanently* affected the developing male brain, a process called "masculinization," while the absence of androgens resulted in undifferentiated or female brains. Henceforward, these originators of femininity and masculinity in sexual and nonsexual behavior were no longer thought to be regulated exclusively by hormones, but to have a *neurological* basis in the brain for long-term effects.

Scientists' acceptance of the organization theory perpetuated the opposition between the concepts of masculinity and femininity in theory and in research practice, although this opposition became asymmetrical. They conceptualized femininity as a condition reflecting the *absence* of androgens. These chemicals ruled male brain development and behavior. We might say that the hormonal opposition or dualist images of masculinity and femininity turned into a neurological monism of masculinity. To describe the situation in Laqueur's terms: A one-sex model came into being. In this way, the theory fit the existing, dual image of gender like a glove, given its emphasis on ideas about masculinity and femininity as formulated by Freud. These ideas associated masculinity with the presence of a penis and femininity with the lack of a penis. In the organization theory, which was studied mainly in animals during this period, masculinity was interpreted as *"presence"* of the "male" hormones in the brain, thereby resulting in sexual initiative and activity. Femininity was interpreted as *"absence"* of the same "male" hormones in the brain, thereby resulting in sexual receptivity and passivity.[5]

Money and Ehrhardt's extension of the theory to humans meant that the presence of androgens before birth became associated with complex issues such as intelligence and career orientation and their absence with a preoccupation for pretty clothes and motherhood.[6] The function of hormones was scientifically translated into prevailing perceptions of masculine and feminine behavior.

1971–1976: Introduction of Femininity, Return to Dualism

In 1971, the period of unhindered production of knowledge based on the organization theory came to an end. The landmark of this period consists of Beach's 1971 publication with its severe criticism of this research. Shortly thereafter, Schoelch-Krieger's demonstration of scientific ignorance of active sexual behavior among female laboratory rats followed.

In general, feminist questions about the origin of femininity and masculinity in behavior diverted attention from the development of male sexual behavior to the development of and differences between masculinity and femininity in behavior. Several new groups joined the network responsible for the acceptance of knowledge about the development of femininity and masculinity in behavior.

The first new group involved in the development of knowledge about the biological background of behavior consisted of women scientists in the field of behavioral neuroendocrinology. For the first time in the history of biomedical sciences, these researchers approached the investigation *as women*. They designed new concepts and methods for studying their questions about active contributions by females in sexual interactions. As a result, they penetrated the masculine circle of research into androgens, male brain development, and behavior, thus making "femininity" perceptible within the prenatal hormone paradigm.

This process met with some resistance among male scientists. During this period, interactions between male and female scientists became constitutive for the development of knowledge based on the organization theory. More specifically, Frank Beach criticized research based on the organization theory in 1971 in an effort to persuade the researchers in the network to return to the biopsychological theory he had formulated in the 1940s. This theory was based on the effects of hormones on sexual and learning experiences in adult life. Beach's critique arose in part from his fear that psychologists would lose their authority. As research based on the organization theory implied a focus on brain development instead of simply on behavior, it became neurological rather than psychological. Beach's efforts toward persuasion, however, were unsuccessful. The researchers of the network continued their research based on the organization theory. Although scientists in the field accepted his criticism to a certain extent, Beach and his collaborators remained isolated in their rejection of the theory that prenatal hormones differentiated brains according to male and female characteristics.

In the years following 1971, women researchers designed several concepts for studying hormonal effects on active female sexual behavior. Beach used the existence of these different concepts as an opportunity to "mend his ways." In 1976, he proposed ideas that unified the existing variety of concepts used to investigate active female sexual behavior. Beach's abandonment of his biopsychological theory was as influential as his proposal of new concepts for developing this field. He submitted that prenatal hormones induced the development of centers in the female brain that control active sexual behavior. By means of this suggestion, Beach thus modified the organization theory. Just as other scientists had previously accepted that the hypothalamus steered male sexual behavior, he proposed that control centers for female sexual behavior also lay in the hypothalamus.

It emerged that Beach offered to abandon his psychological theory (which focused on behavior) in favor of the organization theory (which focused on development of the brain). In return, he was able to resume discussions with "mainstream" scientists adhering to the prenatal hormone paradigm. Metaphorically, Beach negotiated with other scientists about knowledge concerning the development of sexual behavior. Quite possibly, this step was important for renewing Beach's authority as a psychologist in biobehavioral sciences.

It is likely that Beach's conversion was also stimulated by the findings of Money and Ehrhardt (published in 1972) concerning the effects of prenatal hormones on later human behavior. Money and Ehrhardt described prenatal hormones as affecting a variety of human behaviors associated with masculinity and femininity, including career choice and ambitions for motherhood. In fact, Money and Ehrhardt's work mediated the reorganization of perceptions of femininity and masculinity in human behavior based on laboratory practice.

Their work attracted a group to the network that consisted of physicians and psychiatrists practicing in medical fields where the images were actually formed. Physicians and psychiatrists interpreted Money and

Ehrhardt's investigations for use in medical practice; the work served as a partial basis for treatment of pseudohermaphrodites, people born as intersex, and was designed to make them "normal" women and men, both in anatomical and in psychological respects. Physicians and psychiatrists provided psychological counseling and evaluated their surgical and hormonal therapies according to the prescriptive views of femininity and masculinity of behavior in Money and Ehrhardt's investigations into pseudohermaphrodites. Thus, an obligatory point of passage for people seeking medical treatment for their sexual ambiguity emerged from knowledge about the prenatal hormone paradigm.

The feminist psychologists Maccoby and Jacklin also referred to the work of Money and Ehrhardt to support their own findings on psychological differences. In 1974, Maccoby and Jacklin published a book about their research that reduced the long list of psychological sex differences to a few "real" differences in behavior between women and men. The authors suggested that the "real" differences were biological.

It has become clear that the different groups engaged in the network at that time were overwhelmed by biomedical knowledge about prenatal hormones affecting behavior. However, feminist investigators who conducted research from the perspective of behavior as social in origin were also productive and assumed several positions in the network. For example, Sandra Bem, a feminist psychologist, designed a new model for studying masculine and feminine personality characteristics that originated in the feminist debate about androgyny. In her model, which she called orthogonal, femininity and masculinity were no longer regarded as opposites but as independent of each other. Individuals could integrate personality traits perceived as feminine or masculine characteristics in psychological research based on these models.

The behavioral neuroendocrinologist Richard Whalen adapted Bem's orthogonal model for research based on the organization theory. Biomedical scientists subscribing to the prenatal hormone paradigm accepted the concepts of masculinity and femininity as theoretically independent. They had difficulties, however, in accepting the experimental implications of this model, especially in investigations of human behavior. A major objection involved behavioral categories for women and men provided by the results of research based on this model, which conflicted with traditional views of masculinity or femininity in behavior.

Other feminists, for example Beach's student Leonore Tiefer, began to criticize research on prenatal hormone effects on humans for neglecting or underestimating the influence of social mechanisms on the development of masculinity and femininity in behavior. Criticism on this point also arose in the third period. Eventually this led to new approaches in research. For example, Celia Moore developed a research design considering social as well as hormonal factors on behavioral development of rats.

In this second period, the social conditions surrounding the interactions in the network differed markedly from those in the first period. Many disciplines resurrected the nurture versus nature debate. In contrast to the previous period, the origins of femininity and masculinity in behavior became subject to question. Male scientists no longer ruled supreme in the production of knowledge. Female researchers in biomedical sciences and feminist scholars in other disciplines joined the interactions in the network. In this period, first Beach and later feminists as well questioned biologists' competence in the production of knowledge about human behavior. Both Beach's and the feminists' objections to the organization theory were motivated by strategic considerations. Unlike Beach, who became isolated, feminists formed a large group and insisted on providing knowledge about the development of behavior from a perspective that was totally incongruent with that of biomedical scientists.

These conditions were not merely negative for biomedical scientists. Questioning the origin of sex differences also increased general interest in this type of research. The new conditions complicated the acceptance of knowledge based on the prenatal hormone paradigm.

As a result of feminist questions about the origin of femininity and the introduction of oral contraceptives, it became acceptable (and sometimes even compulsory) to include within the prenatal hormone paradigm female sexuality and other characteristics regarded as feminine subjects for investigation.

In this period, an entirely positive condition for acceptance of knowledge based on the prenatal hormone paradigm involved acknowledgment of the value of this knowledge for treating pseudohermaphrodites. This view accorded social legitimation to future investigations and facilitated the acceptance of knowledge produced by biomedical scientists. Under the conditions that had ruled the previous period, Dörner's application of this type of knowledge in "curing" or preventing male homosexuality had been controversial. In this period, more than anything else, physicians' and psychiatrists' adaptation of knowledge for medical practice labeled this knowledge as truth. The possibility of affecting masculinity and femininity in behavior as a result of knowledge based on the prenatal hormone paradigm was considered proof of its accuracy.

The 1970s ushered in a change in the cognitive conditions for acceptance of knowledge about the development of behavior. Biomedical scientists included the effects of estrogens and the female brain in the prenatal hormone paradigm.

After a few years of confusion, biomedical scientists acknowledged that prenatal androgens had to be converted into estrogens before becoming functional in brain development. In the network, this idea gained acceptance after scientists constructed mechanisms that salvaged the idea of a dualist function of sex hormones. Even though androgens had to be converted into estrogens to become active, these hormones continued to be considered responsible for male brain development, while estrogens were ascribed a role in female brain development. Thus, both androgens and estrogens became necessary for development of the brain, and the dualist function ascribed to hormones in brain development became symmetrical.

In their research designs, however, biomedical scientists assigned different meanings to the effects of prenatal sex hormones on the male or the female hypothalamus. They defined the function of estrogens to the extent that they stimulated behavior traditionally viewed as female and attributed the same role to androgens for masculine behavior.

From 1971 to 1976, scientists, physicians, and some feminists subjected the images of masculinity and femininity in accepted knowledge to another radical reconstruction. The masculine monism of androgens, masculinization of the brain, and development of male behavior in the original organization theory turned into a dualism. Estrogens, female brain development, and femininity in behavior became targets of investigation.

In this period, estrogens were assigned new functions in female brain development, which resulted in new meanings of femininity in behavior. The functions ascribed to androgens did not change: These chemicals remained messengers of unchanged meanings of masculinity. The Freudian images of masculinity as a presence and femininity as an absence were replaced by modernized ideas of masculinity and femininity, where femininity was no longer conceptualized as an absence.

1977–1985: Dualism Unlimited

The third period marked the beginning of interference from feminist interactions in the network along with progress in prenatal hormone research in humans. The controversy about the effects of nature or nurture on the development of behavior became increasingly relevant. This period was characterized by the 1977 article published by the biomedical scientists David Quadagno and Robert Briscoe and the feminist sociologist Jill Quadagno. Their article questioned the possibility of investigating the effects of prenatal hormones on human brain development and behavior. During this period, research on prenatal hormone effects on human behavior was illustrated by the problem of distinguishing between the effects of prenatal hormones and those of sociocultural factors on the behavior of humans.

A scientist's loyalty to the prenatal hormone paradigm no longer depended on her or his area of specialization. Some sociologists adhered to the prenatal hormone paradigm in their explanations for differences in behavior between women and men. Some of the scientists who had previously belonged to a discipline that subscribed to the prenatal hormone paradigm openly doubted the feasibility of isolating the "nature" component in human behavioral development from the "nurture" component for investigation purposes. For instance, Robert Briscoe and David Quadagno joined forces with the sociologist Jill Quadagno to play a characteristically unorthodox role in the network. The Dutch psychiatrist Froukje Slijper, who attributed "tomboy" behavior in intersex girls to postnatal factors, also typified this period. In the previous period, psychiatrists had generally subscribed to the prenatal hormone paradigm. Such contributions had weakened the positions of scientists, who explained their results only in terms of prenatal hormone effects. Although their conclusions became more equivocal, scientists investigating prenatal hormone effects in children whose mothers had received hormone treatments during pregnancy extended the implications of prenatal hormone effects to a growing number of behavioral categories.

Psychologists such as Benbow, Stanley, Galaburda, and Geschwind substantiated these findings in their reports about many more types of differences between women and men, for example sex differences in verbal and visual-spatial skills and in aspects of health. They suggested not only that the hypothalami of males and females reflected the influence of prenatal hormones but that the distribution of functions in both hemispheres of the cortex and the connection between the hemispheres of the brain were affected as well.

The new influential groups in the network included journalists popularizing the knowledge produced by biomedical scientists. They presented scientists' hypotheses about relationships between prenatal hormones and later behavior as facts established beyond question in the scientific community.

In this period, the emphasis on the knowledge of human behavioral development acquired an increasing resemblance to the style of assertions about religious or political faith. On the one hand, most scientists attempted to separate nature and nurture effects in behavioral development. Sometimes their optimism was mixed with antifeminist sentiments.[7] Such antifeminism was formulated with striking clarity by the journalists Anne Moir and David Jessel in their book *BrainSex*, in which they accused feminism of frustrating women and men by encouraging them to abandon their natural inclinations.

On the other hand, feminists produced knowledge about social factors affecting human behavior with the conviction that these aspects were necessary for explaining behavioral sex differences between women and men. Their ideas and criticisms finally created an ideological rift between biomedical scientists; some expressed doubts, whereas others considered the prenatal hormone paradigm essential for understanding sexual dimorphism in behavior. In this period, the dominant cultural views of the sexes were still dichotomous, whether they were they biological, cultural (as many feminists asserted), or a combination of the two (as most biomedical scientists believed).

While cognitive conditions for the acceptance of knowledge about the development of behavior did not differ significantly from the second period, ideas about the hormonal influences believed to affect behavior became more complex. As in the previous period, the name of a hormone generally reflected its supposed function in the differentiation of masculinity and femininity in behavior according to scientists' views. Investigations of the effects of many more types of hormones (including synthetic hormones) revealed that some hormones were unruly and could produce androgenic effects in some experiments and anti-androgenic or estrogenic effects in others. Scientists designated this new category of hormones "weak androgens."

During this period, biomedical researchers, both men and women, related explanations for many types of traditional femininity and masculinity in human behavior to the realm of prenatal hormones and attributed sex differences in behavior to differences in brain structure. Feminists also furthered the extension of the dualist images of femininity and masculinity that had evolved in the previous period by opposing the prenatal hormone paradigm in their attempt to attribute the differences in behavior between the sexes to environmental factors.

Although biomedical models since the mid–1970s had offered an opportunity to cross the theoretical boundaries of femininity and masculinity, dualist ideology concerning hormonal function survived. For this reason, the scientific community disputed experimental results on prenatal hormone effects in humans that actually transgressed the boundaries of femininity and masculinity constructed by hormonal functions. Reinisch's findings that the use of prenatal estrogens made children less sensitive and more corteric (more inclined to think than to feel) were largely rejected. Had biomedical scientists accepted the results of this research, they would have undermined the prenatal hormone paradigm completely.

Throughout these three periods, scientists, physicians (both feminists and other individuals), and feminist scholars involved in interactions about the acceptance of knowledge concerning development of behavior generally reinforced dualism in masculinity and femininity. In addition, they changed the meanings of biological masculinity and femininity. Femininity in the brain changed from "undifferentiated" to "located in the hypothalamus" and was acknowledged as a structural principle in the organization of the functions in the brain. After 1959, masculinity in the brain was located in the hypothalamus; it also became accepted as a structural principle in the organization of the brain from the 1980s onward.

The new conditions, which now involved the dynamics of the positions of the distinct groups or individuals and their role in reconstructing images of masculinity and femininity, are more complicated than initial impressions might suggest. During the first period, predominantly male scientists constructed the prenatal hormone paradigm that ascribed the development of male brains and behavior to "male" hormones. In the second period, female and male researchers involved both estrogens and androgens in the development of male and female brains and behavior. In the second and third periods, male and female investigators defined the "androgenity" or "estrogenity" of a hormone according to the extent of its effect on behavioral categories socially regarded as masculine or feminine. Thus, the entrance of female researchers and the rise of feminism seem to have introduced estrogens and femininity into the picture of the prenatal hormone paradigm. By 1970, however (i.e., before many women researchers had entered biomedical science), some scientists had already described the necessity of conversion of androgens to estrogens for their activation in the development of the brain.

The development of behavioral neuroendocrinology involved a complex of factors, including the emergence of the question about the origin of sex differences, the emergence of women researchers, and Beach's method of including the new concepts in his "negotiations." Taken together, these aspects made it possible for biomedical scientists to accept the results of investigations into the effects of prenatal estrogens as differentiating substances in the brain.

1959–1985: Dualism Revised

During this period, dual images of masculinity and femininity had clearly become important enough to be questioned within biomedical science. Obviously, the development of male sexual behavior (especially homosexual behavior) and of sex differences in behavior needed to be elucidated.

A danger inherent in almost all dualistic thought (and certainly in the duality of masculinity and femininity) is that one half of the duality is assigned a superior significance. We have seen that characteristics that are less socially desirable, such as a lower IQ, passivity, and a lack of dominance and aggression (which results in the desire for care rather than the ambition to pursue a career), are ascribed to women and were originally attributed to a lack of "male" hormones before birth. Later, scientists suggested that the structure of the male brain tended to endow men with superior visual-spatial ability. Some used this result to explain men's achievements in technical fields. Women's tendency toward superior verbal skills, however, did not appear to lead to success in politics or other careers in which this skill could be socially acknowledged. Male homosexuality was also seen as a female orientation and implicitly (or sometimes even explicitly) regarded as at variance with the "superior" segment of mankind.

These ideas about masculinity and femininity influenced scientific study during the period of this research, although some people recognized the limitations of the dual images of masculinity and femininity in the 1970s.

In 1974, Whalen proposed independent rather than dualistic concepts of masculinity and femininity. According to this conceptualization, male and female individuals could exhibit both masculine and feminine character traits. At this time, however, the functions scientists ascribed to hormones remained dualistic. Androgens and estrogens retained their roles as chemical messengers of masculinity and femininity, respectively.

In Reinisch's 1977 publication on prenatal hormone effects in humans, she appeared to imply potentiation instead of differentiation of behavior by hormones. At the time, it was not yet possible to replace the differentiation in masculinity and femininity with the potentiation of general human behavior by prenatal hormones. Such a cognitive shift in the function of hormones would have made the organization theory redundant. The idea of the integration of masculine and feminine behavior or character traits had yet to obtain general social acceptance. The femininity-masculinity dualism remained very much alive.

In the 1980s, Whalen was also responsible for recognizing the limitations of the dual function ascribed to hormones. He noted the impact of the presupposed dual effects of hormones on experiments and interpretations when their designations reflected one of the two sexes (such as "androgen" or "estrogen"). He argued: "Testosterone is the most potent natural androgen known for maintaining sexual behavior in castrated males and in many species. But testosterone can also induce those responses characteristic of sexual receptivity in castrated females of several species. . . . These observations suggest that our attribution of a quality to a compound (e.g. defining testosterone as an androgen and not as an estrogen) *reflects an often unstated conviction about mechanism of action*" (emphasis added).[8]

In the late 1980s, however, most researchers studying hormones, brain development, and behavior adhered to the theory, although its validity was questioned on other grounds. For example, it was argued that "differences in mounting behavior between male and female rats can be wholly explained by the different gonadal hormonal milieu in adulthood together with the different external genital anatomy."[9] Others defended the organization theory.[10]

Is it possible to conceive of other courses than the ones actually taken by this field of research? I believe it is justified to argue that if the context had been one in which masculinity and femininity were not regarded as dualistic entities, the organization theory—had it had been proposed at all—would have been different. The extrapolations to nonsexual behavior (so-called "sex-dimorphic" behaviors), which assume a division in behavior between males and females, would probably not have occurred.

Moreover, it seems unlikely that a scientific translation of images of masculinity and femininity in describing the functions of hormones would have occurred had masculinity and femininity not been regarded as dualities within society. "Male" and "female," and "androgenic," "anti-androgenic," and "estrogenic" hormones would probably not have been thought to exist as such, since scientists have observed their emergence and operation at significant levels in both sexes. Within this alternative scenario, the possibility of the conversion of hormones would probably have been proposed earlier. Moreover, if the theory relating to the significance of androgens for the development of sexual and other behavioral characteristics had not been developed, it seems unlikely that the problem of the prevention of masculinization of the female brain would have surfaced. However, the existence of masculinity and femininity in the brain retained the status of an indisputable fact, both in the research based on the organization theory and in the opposition between nature and nurture. Following the incorporation of "the second sex" into the organization theory, the nature-nurture opposition also became increasingly problematic.

Nature-Nurture Revised

Throughout the period covered by this study, feminists, biologists, and many other individuals applied several perspectives to the nurture-nature debate. The issue acquired an increasingly ideological connotation. The proponents of nurture as the only factor in the development of differences in behavior and social positions between the sexes considered the parties who assigned nature a major role in behavioral development to be conservatives. Scientists in this field of research, however, changed their opinion regarding the role of nature. As we saw, social factors gradually gained acceptance as essential for understanding the development of behavior. How did scientists perceive the role of hormones (both before and after birth) in this field of research, and how did their views change during the period covered by this study?

Researchers working with the organization theory assumed that animals and humans were born with male or female brains. Subsequently, social and cultural factors affected these male or female brains in the sense that women had different learning strengths. The final outcome involved differences in behavior between the sexes. Thus, a biological basis that was influenced by social and cultural factors resulted in certain types of behavior or characteristics. Until the early 1980s, this principle formed the foundation of research on the development of the brain and behavior, the so-called *additive* research model:

Nature + Nurture = Behavior

For scientists taking this approach, the 1960s were relatively carefree, especially for researchers studying brain development and adult sexual behavior in animals. They believed their laboratory animals exhibited the same behavior as animals in natural environments, and they were not concerned about possible social influences on observed behaviors. This carefree period ended when critics asserted that parental expectations about the female or male behavior of their offspring, whether human or animal, outweighed hormone effects in understanding the development of behavior of the sexes. This criticism made sense to many investigators of behavioral development. Most studies were performed with children or animals with ambiguous genitals, but ambiguous parental expectations about male or female behavior were not taken into consideration.

Researchers tried to define this factor by studying the effects of prenatal hormones on humans in another group: DES children endowed with normal genitals. Their mothers had taken hormones during pregnancy that supposedly affected the brains and behavioral development of their children. Researchers tried to consider all kinds of social factors in establishing the effects of prenatal hormones on the behaviors they registered. The impact of social background, education, medical history, and the like was determined by conducting similar examinations on control groups. These effects on their behavior were subtracted from the total, and the remainder was considered the effect of the hormones taken by their mothers during pregnancy. As this procedure did not successfully rule out prenatal hormone effects, scientists regarded this problem as a drawback of the additive model. They called for an interactive or biosocial model in this type of research.

An *interactive* model is based on the assumption that development of behavior results from a combination of biological factors and social environment:

$$\text{nature} \rightleftarrows \text{nurture} \rightarrow \text{behavior}$$

The interactive approach assigns biological and social factors the same meaning in the development of behavior and seems to erase the opposition between nature and nurture. Both elements receive equal representation in this model. An interactive model does not emphasize either component. In prenatal hormone studies, however, there is a snake in the grass. The hormones are active before birth, a period during which the role of social influences is obviously minimal. Moreover, researchers realized they could not possibly investigate all factors in behavioral development. Therefore, they abandoned their efforts to isolate a single factor as the cause of a particular behavior. Nowadays, researchers mention a coherence or correlation between the occurrence of phenomena, although their wish to find a causal relationship remains. Moreover, research has been forced to acknowledge that, in principle, interacting elements can be studied separately. By definition, research involves ordering and classifying information, but classifying the factors that influence behavior is not limited to one study or even one research institute. The interacting elements, which roughly include "the biological" and "the social," are spread over several disciplines, and this breakdown has major consequences for our views of all kinds of phenomena. Whether a concept or an entity is designated as biological or social is in part the result of academic division into disciplines.

For example, depression is considered to result from an interaction between biological processes in the brain and the social circumstances of the individual concerned. These interactive factors are distinguished according to the disciplines. Biomedical laboratory research focuses on processes in the brain, and psychological studies examine life experiences and coping strategies. Researchers in both fields can refer to each other's work, but the differences in disciplinary approaches suggest that depression is caused either by individual biology or by difficult social circumstances rather than by a combination of the two. Treatment reflects the different causes of the interaction: Biomedical scientists have developed antidepressants and psychologists have designed psychotherapy. In the first case, depression is considered a physical illness; in the second, it is regarded as an emotional ailment. Actually, this distinction is far more rigidly maintained for other diseases, such as migraine or chronic fatigue syndrome (a relatively recently defined disease), than for depression. Depression is often treated with a combination of drugs and therapy, referring to both causes.

Aside from the difficulty of isolating causes in interactive factors, another drawback of research based on interaction models is that sex differences in behavior or other phenomena are considered to be the outcome, just as in the additive model. Instead of presenting the sum of an addition, the model becomes the result of interaction by social and biological variables. Results of research to establish information about those interactions seem to congeal at the moment of investigation and are presented as factual evidence.

An interactionist research model thus seems to be a more faithful representation of behavioral development than an additive model. Research based on both models, however, represents behavior as the final result of biological and social circumstances. In addition, recent studies have examined the effects of behavior on human physiology. For example, training affects muscular development and, as most women know, stress influences menstrual periods. The question is whether our brains can adapt to our behavior. If so, what model would provide an understanding of such developments?

Behavior Changes Nature and Nurture

Within certain limits, the body adapts to behavior. How does this ability affect differences in opportunities for women and men? Susan Ward and Brian Whipp published remarkable findings on this subject. They reviewed world marathon records since the beginning of the twentieth century. Their question as to whether marathon runners would ever reach a maximum speed led them to investigate the decrease in running times. Remarkably, they noted a consistent decrease in the difference between male and female running times since the 1950s. From their extrapolation of the decreasing difference, Ward and Whipp predicted that a woman marathon runner would equal the record of her male counterpart before the end of the twentieth century.[11] The realization of this scenario will remain a subject of uncertainty for a few more years. Nevertheless, the *International Herald Tribune* considered this finding worthy of publication on the front page on January 3, 1992.[12] Until recently, it was thought that muscle development and female body structure put women at such a disadvantage that they would never be able to run as fast as men. While the study deals with outstanding results from athletes with intensive training, this finding is most remarkable, considering existing cultural beliefs about the biological possibilities and constraints for women and men. In this case, it seems justified to conclude that physiology is more adaptable than we could ever have imagined.[13]

Such reports, together with television programs about female athletes, have changed expectations of the possibilities for women and men and have had a clear impact on actual achievements. In 1955, women who aspired to run the marathon were the exception. Over the years, such ambitions have become increasingly commonplace. Growing numbers of women participate in sports such as cycle racing, ice skating, and sailing. Not long ago, the recent achievements in these sports were considered impossible. The response "that's not for girls" to women's desire to excel in sports is obsolete. The fact that women started training (behavior) thus influenced both their individual physiology (biology, i.e., nature) and parental expectations about their daughters' abilities (nurture).

The course of events at the beginning of this century was comparable. Notwithstanding the general idea (based on "scientific" results) that women were too vulnerable or lacked the intelligence for academic studies, women matriculated at universities and exhibited academic achievements that were certainly equal to those of their male counterparts. As a consequence, general views of women's intellectual capacities changed, along with the unflattering scientific underpinnings of those views.

Another example attests to behavioral modifications as a result of a changing environment. In evaluating differences between the sexes in verbal and spatial skills, Janet Hyde noted a trend of convergence over the past twenty-five years.[14] She related this process to the opportunities for girls and boys, which grew more similar during this period. Hyde does not deny that the brain plays a role in these skills. On the contrary, it coordinates all behavior. Hyde believes these decreasing differences reflect the brain's adaptation to changing educational and social opportunities for boys and girls. These examples demonstrate that some types of behavior and skill are not the final result of an interaction between biology (the brain) and environment. Rather, behavior is an agent in this interaction:

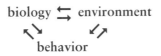

This *transformative* model depicts the interaction between biology, environment, and behavior. This model can enhance the insights into the development of individual behavior that we have derived from the interactive model. It requires a different methodology, however, than is usually applied in experiments. This model also has implications for the conceptualization of sex and gender in feminist theory. The scheme above can be presented as follows:

$$\text{nature (sex)} \leftrightarrows \text{nurture (environment)}$$
$$\searrow \quad \nearrow$$
$$\text{gender (femininity or masculinity)}$$

Prior to a more detailed discussion of this model, I will present additional supporting arguments in favor of this model, which actually proposes abandoning the static sex-gender distinction.

Feminism Revised

How do the results of this study affect the feminist distinction between sex and gender? To date, feminist research has focused mainly on the social phenomena constructing gender (i.e., femininity). Many feminist scholars labeled biological knowledge about sex extraneous to their interests. Generally, feminists considered biology to be a discipline providing knowledge irrelevant for social change. Ironically, as biomedical scientists increased their efforts to avoid external influences, feminism propagated the idea of innate factors for femininity or masculinity in the brain and behavior. Questions about the development of female sexual behavior and the search for "real" psychological differences between women and men proved constitutive for the biological dichotomy in female and male brains and behavior. Probably, many feminists neither expected nor wanted this result.

Women researchers and feminists who participated in the network also affected the production of knowledge.[15] Their questions inspired by feminism made "femininity" visible and turned it into a subject of investigation. New concepts emerged and existing ones changed. These women accepted the presupposition of a truth about the biological backgrounds of sex differences that could be revealed with scientific methods.

Other researchers doubted the results of the biological research into sex differentiation in the brain. They criticized the methodology used and influenced the production of knowledge in the network. Texts criticizing research methods of investigation into prenatal hormone effects in animals and humans had a major impact and culminated in a call for a biosocial research perspective. These publications provided opportunities for different research questions and consequently different results as well. For example, Slijper's findings revealed that parents' uncertainty concerning their child's sex and the view that intersex children receiving medical treatment are ill can affect their behavior more than prenatal hormones.

Is criticism of methodology therefore necessary to escape biological determinism? Although criticizing methodology can yield valuable results, I would rather suggest changing the feminist evaluation of biological and social factors affecting the development of behavior.

This study has demonstrated the role of cultural context in neuroendocrinological investigations. Sex proves not to be an unquestionable and objective physical characteristic. Since 1959, the scientific location of sex has traveled from the genitals through the chemicals these organs produce (hormones) to the brain. Historically, therefore, sex is not a fixed category. In thirty years, the significance of sex has changed according to the context. Medical practice labeled the universal nature of this meaning of sex as truth.

Like gender characteristics, biological sex is thus ascribed a meaning that varies according to time and place and according to whether researchers choose sex or gender as the subject of their investigation. As we saw, scientists in behavioral neuroendocrinology struggled as much as feminists with the distinction between sex and gender. Question arises concerning the basis that remains for the feminist distinction between sex and gender and the distinction between biological and social aspects.

I suggest abandoning these dualities by conducting research based on the transformative model. Lynda Birke, who originally proposed this model,[16] has presented more biological arguments to substantiate that not only biological and environmental factors (resulting in certain behavioral characteristics) interact, but that behavior itself is part of these interactions. The model suggests regarding biology, environment, and behavior as three interactive factors. In this model of gender, characteristics considered masculine or feminine are not dependent variables of an interaction between social and biological factors. Rather than being a fixed individual property, gender is part of these interactive processes. According to Birke: "Adult gender identity, as woman or as man, can only be understood as the present dynamic point in a continually evolving process which includes the real lived experience of our biological selves as well as the social meaning and economic context of our lives."[17]

This model transforms the sex-gender duality into a dynamic understanding of people's behavior and identity. Gender identity is no longer a static attribute of individuals. Gender undergoes a lifetime of reconstruction to reflect social and biological events, such as menstruation, sexual activity, childbirth, and parenthood, or the absence of any of these experiences. Gender reconstruction among individuals eventually changes the meanings of social and biological experiences. For example, while masculinity ("being a man") formerly implied a career, it has also come to include parenthood and responsibilities for child care in some cases. Viewing sex and gender as interactive entities is also of strategic value. Considering them to be dynamic invokes change more easily than conceptualizing them as static.

This perception of sex and gender allows us to admit to experiencing our biological being, while seeing it as embedded in complex, interactive operations. These processes can undergo transformation both during the lifetime of an individual and between individuals over the course of history, as the social and historical contexts of individual lives change. Neither biological factors nor social environment alone determine any aspect of our behavior or our skills.[18]

Science and Gender Perspectives

This study describes the influence of groups involved in the interaction on acceptance of knowledge in the network. I therefore recommend that women (or scientists with a feminist identity) enter the scientific networks in which knowledge is produced and accepted and the circles that apply this knowledge in medical practice. It is important that women in these positions obtain an opportunity to formulate their own research questions and to design methods for investigating these questions. New results will facilitate the development of new methods of treatment.

In the Netherlands, women are still underrepresented in research carried out at biology faculties. These departments are launching affirmative action programs, both to provide women with equal opportunities for careers in science and as a means of developing more balanced knowledge.[19]

Organizational structures and laboratory practices are products of social and historical processes.[20] In the 1970s, the widespread emergence of women researchers was a milestone in the history of science. Although transforming these bastions will be difficult, I believe they may reflect equal representation of women in science in the future. Over the past twenty years, the rise of women's studies in many university faculties and women's health organizations has exemplified the change in organizational structures that has culminated in different cognitive approaches. As for the disciplinary traditions mentioned above, epistemological and methodological issues have been questioned in women's studies.[21] In women's health organizations, for example, premenstrual, menstrual, and menopausal complaints are no longer defined solely as personal problems with "changing hormones" but also as conditions reflecting the social perception of femininity and elderly women.

This case study on the development of research based on the organization theory highlights the importance of ideas about masculinity and femininity in the production of knowledge. Previously, feminist scholars demonstrated that this field of biology was not the only field affected by these ideas. Ruth Hubbard described the effect of ideas about masculinity and femininity on evolutionary biology in her article, "Have Only Men Evolved?"[22] Other feminist authors have suggested that the current theory either neglects or underestimates the role of women in evolution. Still other scholars have criticized the mechanisms believed to underlie evolutionary processes.[23] Elaine Morgan and others have developed alternative theories for the evolution of mankind based on the same facts as the current theory about this subject.[24] In these theories, man-the-hunter makes way for woman-the-gatherer as the point of impact of evolutionary processes. These alternative theories made clear that interpretation of facts depends largely on scientists' presuppositions.[25] Possibly, integration of traditional and new concepts will lead to more balanced knowledge.

Nowadays, scientists in a multitude of disciplines derive their theoretical basis, to a certain extent, from knowledge about the evolution of humans. Ruth Bleier lists primate anatomy and physiology, animal sociology (ethology,) physical anthropology and paleontology (the study of variations in structure and function and the correlations between them among humans, other primates, and fossil remains), comparative psychology or psychobiology (across species), sexual and reproductive physiology, population genetics, evolutionary and ecological field biology, and social and cultural anthropology.[26] Thus, analysis in large fields of knowledge can begin with the question: To what extent did images of masculinity and femininity or notions associated with those images play a role in the production of knowledge?

Scientists should therefore discuss the impact on research of ideas associated with masculinity and femininity in order to produce more balanced knowledge. More importantly, students, the future generation of scientists, must become acquainted with the role of views associated with masculinity and femininity in research.

In this study, we have observed that editors of scientific journals and journalists popularizing science function as gatekeepers for the acceptance of new ideas in science and society.[27] Therefore, I recommend that feminists enter this branch of the network in order to influence the acceptance of knowledge.

The conclusion that social images of masculinity and femininity affect the cognitive development of science is relevant for future research. To date, most feminist accounts of gendered science have usually ascribed this condition to the traditional role of men in asking the questions. This study reveals that men are only partly responsible and that the relation between science and sex is far more complex than previous studies had suggested. Social and cultural images of masculinity and femininity and social conditions in science affect the content of science and vice versa. Nevertheless, this interaction does not eliminate the possibility of a relationship between individual scientists and cultural images of masculinity and femininity.

Analyzing the correlation between social conditions and cognitive development in science has emerged as a powerful instrument in changing the relationship between sex and science. It provides knowledge of social and cognitive conditions that may be affected by change. Scientists can question the relation between the historical context and the construction of a scientific theory or concept and the extent of its current application in science. This study has revealed that scientific concepts vary in a changing historical context. In the context of feminism, new questions about the development of female sexual behavior transferred the location of the essence of femininity from female reproductive organs through "female" hormones to "neurological" femininity during the 1970s. In the 1990s, this transformation appears to facilitate explanations of differences in skills between women and men. Questions about scientific concepts and theories about sex make it possible to place these allegations, which were previously taken for granted, in the context of their era. Obstacles to other conceptual transformations have also been discussed; for example, the question of why Reinisch's results were slow to become accepted uncovered social as well as scientific constraints, which may be overcome in the future.

It is important to analyze the uses of scientific output in specific medical contexts. How is fundamental knowledge used, and how does it function or become accepted as truth in the treatments for individuals? This study has shown that absolute masculinity and femininity do not exist but that these categories are constructed as truths about bodies and psychological characteristics ascribed to females and males. The same interpretation is possible for other features linked to masculinity and femininity, such as fertility or certain illnesses.[28] Insight into the generally accepted status of social images of masculinity and femininity in medical practice and related institutions, such as pharmaceutical industries, is politically important, as it provides ideas for changing these practices.

Thus, it seems useful to analyze the effect of social images about women and men on modern reproductive technologies and hormonal treatments for contraceptive purposes, premenstrual syndrome, and menopause. It might be worthwhile to consider these images in investigations of different practices with regard to prescription of tranquilizers and antidepressants for women and men.

I would also suggest that feminists' scientific interest in "masculinity" might reconstruct this concept and contribute to the "equalization" of the sexes. Sample questions might be: "What were the social and cognitive constraints against the development of contraceptives for men?" and

"Why did male sterility fail to culminate in the development of a treatment for unwanted male sterility?"

Such analyses, as well as experimental laboratory investigations, will further the deconstruction of images of femininity and masculinity. These studies will contribute to the liberation of women and men from such cultural constraints and will result in access to all of the human possibilities in daily life.

1. Femininity and Women in Biology and Feminist Theory

1. See the following: Ruth Hubbard and Marian Lowe, eds., *Genes and Gender,* vols. 1 and 2 (New York: Gordian Press, 1978). Elizabeth Fee, "Nineteenth Century Craniology: The Study of the Female Skull," *Bulletin of the History of Medicine,* 53 (1979), 415–33. Donna Haraway, "In the Beginning Was the Word: The Genesis of Biological Theory," *Signs: Journal of Women in Culture and Society,* 6, no. 3 (1981). Ruth Hubbard, "Have Only Men Evolved," in S. Harding and M. B. Hintikka, eds., *Discovering Reality: Feminist Perspectives on Epistemology, Metaphysics, Methodology and Philosophy of Science* (Dordrecht: Reidel, 1983). Ruth Bleier, *Science and Gender: A Critique of Biology and Its Theories on Women* (New York: Pergamon, 1984). Anne Fausto-Sterling, *Myths of Gender: Biological Theories on Women and Men* (New York: Basic, 1985). Lynda Birke, *Women, Feminism and Biology: The Feminist Challenge* (Brighton: Harvester, 1986).

2. Judith Butler, *Gender Trouble: Feminism and the Subversion of Identity* (New York: Routledge, 1990), p. 7.

3. Thomas Laqueur, *Making Sex: Body and Gender from the Greeks to Freud* (Cambridge: Harvard University Press, 1990), p. 12.

4. Ibid., p. 8.

5. Laqueur portrays the sexes in the one-sex model as hierarchical, while in the two-sex model the sexes are different. Descriptions of differences have become possible only recently, even though the hierarchy of the sexes has persisted. Current anatomy texts always discuss the development or functions of male parts before female ones.

6. Laqueur, *Making Sex,* p. 154.

7. Anne Fausto-Sterling, "The Five Sexes: Why Male and Female Are Not Enough," *The Sciences* (March-April 1993), 20–24.

8. Michel Foucault, *Herculine Barbin, dite Alexina B. presenté par Michel Foucault* (Paris: Gallimard, 1978). The Dutch translation of Barbine's memoirs includes an introduction by Foucault: Herculine Barbin, *Mijn herinneringen* (Amsterdam: Arbeiderspers, 1982). Foucault suggests that this use of the medical term "pseudo" entails the existence of an underlying real male or female to be discovered by medical examination.

9. Foucault brought the existence and the experiences of a pseudo-hermaphrodite to the attention of a larger public by publishing *Herculine Barbin, dite Alexina B.* See also Michel Foucault, *The History of Sexuality* (New York: Vintage, 1980 [*Histoire de la sexualité* 1. *La volonté de savoir* (Paris: Gallimard, 1976)]).

10. Butler, *Gender Trouble.*

11. Stefan Hirschauer, "The Manufacture of Bodies in Surgery," *Social Studies of Science,* 21 (1991), 279–319.

12. Simone de Beauvoir, *The Second Sex,* trans. H. M. Parshley (New York: Knopf, 1953).

13. Charles H. Phoenix, Roger W. Goy, Arnold A. Gerall, and William C. Young, "Organization Action of Testosterone Propionate on the Tissues Mediating Mating Behaviors in the Female Guinea Pig," *Endocrinology,* 65 (1959), 369–82.

14. John Money and Anke A. Ehrhardt, *Man and Woman, Boy and Girl: Differentiation and Dimorphism of Gender Identity from Conception to Maturity* (Baltimore: Johns Hopkins University Press, 1972). A. W. H. Buffery and J. A. Gray, "Sex Differences in the Development of Spatial and Linguistic Skills," in C. Onsted and D. C. Taylor, eds., *Gender Differences: Their Onthogeny and Significance* (London: Churchill Livingstone, 1975).

15. Anne Moir and David Jessel, *BrainSex: The Real Difference between Men and Women* (London: Michael Joseph, 1989).

16. Hilary Rose and Steven Rose, "On Oppositions to Reductionism," in Dialectics of Biology Group, ed., *Against Biological Determinism* (London: Allison and Busby, 1982), pp. 50–59; Richard Lewontin, Steven Rose, and Leon Kamin, *Not in Our Genes: Biology, Ideology and Human Nature* (New York: Pantheon, 1984).

The feminist strategy of rejecting the competence of biomedical sciences to provide knowledge about sex differences in behavior is questioned by Annemarie Mol, "Baarmoeders, pigment en pyramiden: Over de vraag of anti-racisten en feministen er goed aan doen 'de biologie' haar plaats te wijzen," *Tijdschrift voor vrouwenstudies*, 35 (1988), 276–90.

17. Margaret Mead, *Sex and Temperament in Three Primitive Societies* (New York: Morrow, 1935).

18. Ibid., p. 279.

19. Ibid., p. 280.

20. Margaret Mead, *Coming of Age in Samoa* (New York: Morrow, 1928).

21. Margaret Mead, *Coming of Age* (New York: Mentor, 1949), p. 117.

22. P. Kloos, "De aanval op Margaret Mead," *Intermediair*, 19, no. 28 (July 15, 1983); P. Reeves Sanday, "Margaret Mead's View on Sex Roles in Her Own and Other Societies," *American Anthropologist*, 82, no. 2 (1980), 340–48.

23. D. Freeman, *Mead and Samoa: The Making and Unmaking of an Anthropological Myth* (Cambridge: Harvard University Press, 1983).

24. In her book *Male and Female: A Study of the Sexes in a Changing World* (New York: Morrow, 1949), Mead focused on the biological basis for differences between women and men. This was criticized by Sanday (1980) from a feminist perspective. See also Ina Keuper, "Margaret Mead: Culturele en biologische factoren in de genusverhoudingen," *Nieuwsbrief Landelijk Overleg Vrouwenstudies in de Anthropologie*, 11, no. 2 (1990), 25–40.

25. P. Kloos, *Door het oog van de anthropoloog: Botsende visies bij heronderzoek* (Muiderberg: Coutinho, 1988), pp. 83–95.

In the Netherlands, Professor Buikhuizen's work was very controversial because he started investigations during the early 1970s into biological factors that might possibly lead to criminality. He dropped his study and left academia.

26. Rhoda Kesler Unger, "Through the Looking Glass: No Wonderland Yet! (The Reciprocal Relationship between Methodology and Models of Reality)," *Psychology of Women Quarterly*, 8, no. 1 (1983), 9–33.

27. Bruno Latour, "Give Me a Laboratory and I Will Raise the World," in Karin Knorr and Michael Mulkay, eds., *Science Observed: Perspectives on the Social Studies of Science* (London: Sage, 1983), pp. 141–71.

28. Money and Ehrhardt, *Man and Woman*.

29. Ronald S. Burt, *Toward a Structural Theory of Action* (New York: Academic, 1982).

30. The designation "cultural feminism" was chosen by Alice Echols: "The New Feminism of Yin and Yang," in Ann Snitow, Christine Stansell, and Sharon Thompson, eds., *Powers of Desire: The Politics of Sexuality* (New York: Monthly

Review Press, 1983), pp. 439–59. Cultural feminism equates "women's liberation with the development and preservation of a female counter culture" (p. 441). Adrienne Rich (her early work) and Mary Daly are the best-known feminists in this movement.

31. For more examples, see Ann Oakley, *Subject Women* (New York: Pantheon, 1981). Not all cultural feminists adhered to the view that the differences are of a biological nature. For example, Janice Raymond argues: "Yet there are differences, and some feminists have come to realize that those differences are important whether they spring from socialization, from biology or from the total history of existing as a woman in a patriarchal society" (as quoted in Echols, "The New Feminism of Yin and Yang").

32. For a feminist discussion of essentialism, see a volume titled "The Essential Difference: Another Look at Essentialism," *Differences: A Journal of Feminist Cultural Studies*, 1 (1989).

33. See, for example, Fee, "Nineteenth Century Craniology."

34. In this study I will use "femininity" and "masculinity," "female" and "male" primarily according to this distinction. This study is, however, concerned with biological factors affecting "femininity" and "masculinity" in the behavior of animals and humans, and some descriptions may therefore deviate from the rule.

35. The core of dual concepts of masculinity and femininity found its origin in the traditional division of labor. Masculinity was associated with ambition, dominance, intelligence, independence, assertiveness, aggression, hardiness, rationality. Femininity was associated with nurturing, subordination, intuition, dependence, compassion, unselfishness, sensitivity, and emotionality. Most of these characteristics were thought to be developed in males and females in an oppositional fashion.

36. For an overview of the discussion, see Mary Vetterling-Braggin, ed., *"Femininity," "Masculinity" and "Androgyny": A Modern Philosophical Discussion* (Totowa, N.J.: Littlefield Adams, 1982). The authors deal with the central question of whether the "masculine" is male-linked and the "feminine" is female-linked with respect both to psychological characteristics and social and labor roles. Various notions of sex and gender in the literature are discussed and tested, and methodological difficulties confirming a presupposed sex-gender link are examined. A substantial portion of the book is devoted to the pros and cons of androgyny.

37. Linda Alcoff, "Cultural Feminism versus Post-Structuralism: The Identity Crisis in Feminist Theory," *Signs: Journal of Women in Culture and Society*, 13, no. 31 (1988), 405–36.

38. For an overview of debates in Women's Studies in the Netherlands, see Margo Brouns, *Veertien jaar vrouwenstudies in Nederland* (The Hague: Ministerie van Onderwijs en Wetenschappen, 1988).

39. Alcoff, "Cultural Feminism."

40. Frances B. McCrea and Gerald E. Markle, "The Estrogen Replacement Controversy in the USA and UK: Different Answers to the Same Question?" *Social Studies of Science*, 14 (1984), 1–26.

41. I regard this group of women scientists as feminists. Whether they considered themselves feminists or not is not always clear in their publications.

42. Unger ("Through the Looking Glass") and Evelyn Fox Keller argued that feminist researchers also share the assumptions of the subdisciplines in which they are socialized; see Evelyn Fox Keller, *Reflections on Gender and Science* (New Haven: Yale University Press, 1985).

43. See, for example, Dorothy Price, "Feedback Control of Gonadal and Hypophyseal Hormones: Evolution of the Concept," in Joseph Meites, Bernal T. Donovan, and Samuel M. McCann, eds., *Pioneers in Neuroendocrinology* (New York: Plenum, 1975), pp. 219–39. For womens' position in science, see also Keller, *Reflections on Gender and Science*.

44. The Frankfurt School includes Jürgen Habermas, Herbert Marcuse, and Theodor W. Adorno. See Foucault's, *History of Sexuality*. Foucault argues that desire and power are the main agents in scientific discourse. Bodies of knowledge represent discourses that reflect, express, and generate relations of power. Scientific rules determine the speakers and the content and manner of the discussion, as well as the questions that are permitted and the establishment of what is "true" or "false." Thus, while science appears to be the *uncovering* of truth, it rests upon and conceals the struggle between those who have the power of discourse and those who do not. Both by their practices of exclusion and their definitions of discussion content and perceptions of what is true or false, discourses *produce* rather than reveal truth. The conditions under which the discourses take place reflect conditions of social power at the time and thus themselves define the theories and practices (such as the scientific methodology) brought to bear in the discourse and consequently determine the outcome.

45. Janet Sayers, *Biological Politics, Feminist and Anti-Feminist Perspectives* (London: Tavistock, 1982). Other arguments put forward to keep women away from intellectual activities were that it would decrease their ability to bear children or their breast development.

46. See Hubbard, "Have Only Men Evolved"; Bleier, *Science and Gender,"* esp. chap. 7; Fausto-Sterling, *Myths of Gender*, and Birke, *Women, Feminism and Biology*.

47. Helen Longino and Ruth Doel, "Body, Bias, and Behavior: A Comparative Analysis of Reasoning in Two Areas of Biological Science," *Signs: Journal of Women in Culture and Society*, 9, no. 2 (1983), 207–27.

48. Fausto-Sterling, *Myths of Gender*, p. 9.

49. Germaine Greer, *The Female Eunuch* (London: MacGibbon and Kee, 1970).

50. D. F. Swaab and M. A. Hofman, "Sexual Differentiation of the Human Brain: A Historical Perspective," *Progress in Brain Research*, 61 (1984), 361–75. On page 367 they write: "It seems plausible to suppose that intelligence is determined in part by the amount of brain tissue in excess of that required for receiving sensory information and controlling muscle movements."

51. Sandra Harding, *The Science Question in Feminism* (Ithaca: Cornell University Press, 1986), p. 100.

52. Keller, *Reflections on Gender and Science*.

53. Ibid., esp. part 3: "Theory, Practice and Ideology in the Making of Science."

54. Bleier, *Science and Gender*, p. 200.

55. Helen Longino, *Science as Social Knowledge: Values and Objectivity in Scientific Inquiry* (Princeton: Princeton University Press, 1990), p. 171.

56. Barbara Fried, "Boys Will Be Boys Will Be Boys: The Language of Sex and Gender," in Ruth Hubbard, M. S. Henifin, and B. Fried, eds., *Women Look at Biology Looking at Women* (Cambridge: Schenkman, 1979). Barbara Fried described the act and the consequences of presenting masculinity and femininity as dualism, as mutually exclusive categories in scientific language.

57. In this study I do not distinguish between "right" or "wrong" science.

While such a distinction is possible from a modern feminist perspective, it could also be considered an example of Whig history. I have chosen to describe the origin of the research based on the organization theory as a normal development in science, as "science as usual." Sandra Harding considers this position suitable for analyzing the regularities and underlying causal tendencies in the relationship between science and other social issues, for example, those concerning masculinity and femininity. See Sandra Harding, "How the Women's Movement Benefits Science: Two Views," *Women's Studies International Forum*, 12, no. 3 (1989), 271–83.

58. Londa Schiebinger, "Skeletons in the Closet: The First Illustrations of the Female Skeleton in the 19th-century Anatomy," *Representations*, 14 (1986), 42–83.

59. Ludmilla Jordanova, *Sexual Visions: Images of Gender in Science and Medicine between the Eighteenth and Twentieth Centuries* (Madison: University of Wisconsin Press, 1989).

60. Donna Haraway, "The Contest for Primate Nature: Daughters of Man the Hunter in the Field, 1960–1980," in M. Kann, ed., *The Future of American Democracy* (Philadelphia: Temple University Press, 1983), pp. 175–207; and Donna Haraway, "Situated Knowledges: The Science Question in Feminism and the Privilege of Partial Perspective," *Feminist Studies*, 14, no. 3 (1988), 575–99.

61. Susan E. Bell, "A New Model of Medical Technology Development: A Case Study of DES," *Research in the Sociology of Health Care*, 4 (1986), 1–33; and idem, "Changing Ideas: The Medicalization of Menopause," *Social Science and Medicine*, 24 (1987), 535–42.

62. The first laboratory studies were performed by Bruno Latour and Steve Woolgar; see *Laboratory Life: The Social Construction of Scientific Facts* (Beverly Hills: Sage, 1979); see also Bruno Latour, *Science in Action: How to Follow Scientists and Engineers through Society* (Milton Keynes: Open University Press, 1987).

63. Nelly Oudshoorn, *Beyond the Natural Body: An Archeology of Sex Hormones* (London: Routledge, 1994).

64. Thomas Kuhn, *The Structure of Scientific Revolutions* (Chicago: University of Chicago Press, 1970).

65. Gianna Pomata, "De geschiedenis van vrouwen: een kwestie van grenzen," *Socialistisch Feministische Teksten*, 10 (1987), 61–113.

2. Acceptance of Scientific Theories and Images of Masculinity and Femininity

1. Charles H. Phoenix, Roger W. Goy, Arnold A. Gerall, and William C. Young, "Organization Action of Testosterone Propionate on the Tissues Mediating Mating Behavior in the Female Guinea Pig," *Endocrinology*, 65 (1959), 369–82.

2. Evelyn Fox Keller, *Reflections on Gender and Science* (New Haven: Yale University Press, 1985), and *A Feeling for the Organism: The Life and Work of Barbara McClintock* (New York: Freeman, 1983). Keller argues that scientific theories that agree with existing images of masculinity and femininity are more easily accepted in science than those that deviate from conventional views.

3. Robert W. Goy, "William Caldwell Young, 1899–1965," in J. Meites, B. T. Donovan, and S. McCann, eds., *Pioneers in Neuroendocrinology* (New York: Plenum, 1975), pp. 5–11.

4. Frank A. Beach, "Historical Origins of Modern Research on Hormones and

Behavior," *Hormones and Behavior,* 15 (1981), 325–76. Organization is a concept originating in embryology; it refers to differentiation of organs, starting with the organization of cells.

5. An organizational effect in this case means an effect on the anatomical structure of brain tissues; an activational effect means a temporary effect on the physiology of the tissues.

6. Phoenix et al., "Organization Action," p. 379.

7. Beach, "Historical Origins," p. 350.

8. As cited in Phoenix et al., "Organization Action."

9. Ibid., p. 370.

10. Alfred Jost, "Hormonal Influences in the Development of the Fetus," *Cold Spring Harbor Symposium on Quantitative Biology,* 19 (1964), 167–81.

11. Ruth Bleier, *Science and Gender: A Critique of Biology and Its Theories on Women* (New York: Pergamon, 1984), chap. 4.

12. Interview with Pieter v.d. Schoot and Koos Slob, Department of Physiology, Erasmus University, Rotterdam, April 18, 1988. John Money named this principle in *Love and Love Sickness: The Science of Sex, Gender Difference, and Pair-Bonding* (Baltimore: Johns Hopkins University Press, 1980): "The principle involved, nicknamed the Adam Principle, is the same as governs the differentiation of the genital anatomy, namely, that to differentiate a male something must be added" (p. 5).

13. Articles on this subject have appeared, for example, in *Journal of Comparative and Psychological Psychology, Journal of Reproduction and Fertility, Endocrinology,* and *Journal of Endocrinology.* These journals already existed in the 1960s. During the 1970s several journals were founded in which experimental results concerning biological factors in behaviors were published. One such journal is *Hormones and Behavior.*

14. Before 1964 some authors referred to the organization theory as a hypothesis, or they used phrases such as "the organization theory *suggests. . . ,*" or "it has been reasonably clear that androgens. . . ." In these articles the authors also provided evidence of the validity of the organization theory for the behavior of other animals than guinea pigs; see, for example, R. E. Whalen and R. D. Nadler, "Suppression of the Development of Female Mating Behavior by Estrogen Administered in Infancy," *Science,* 141 (1963), 273–74.

As early as 1963 some authors were using the word "concept," for example, Roger A. Gorski, "Modification of Ovulatory Mechanisms by Postnatal Administration of Estrogen to the Rat," *American Journal of Physiology,* 205 (1963), 842–44.

I view the extension of the theory's validity to nonsexual types of behavior by many authors as the moment when the hypothesis about the organization of the brain by gonadal hormones was accepted in the field as a theory. From this time onward, the organization theory could *predict* the effects of hormones on sexual behavior and was used to *hypothesize* about questions concerning other behavior. See also Chris Boers, *Wetenschap, techniek en samenleving: Bouwstenen voor een kritische wetenschapstheorie* (Meppel: Boom, 1981), pp. 59–65.

15. William C. Young, Robert W. Goy, and Charles H. Phoenix, "Hormones and Sexual Behavior: Broad Relationships Exist between the Gonadal Hormones and Behavior," *Science,* 143 (1964), 212–18.

16. Robert Goy, written interview, August 16, 1988.

17. Young et al., "Hormones and Sexual Behavior," p. 212.

18. For a review of sex differences in rats with respect to sexual and nonsexual behavior, see Huib van Dis and Nanne E. v.d. Poll, "Sexual Differentiation of

Behavior in Rats," *Progress in Brain Research*, 41 (1974), 321–31. According to these authors, nonsexual behaviors have been investigated since 1964.

19. Robert Goy and Bruce McEwen, *Sexual Differentiation of the Brain: Based on a Work Session of the Neurosciences Program* (Cambridge: MIT Press, 1980), pp. 20, 21, 22. On these pages the experimental results of research on the organizing action of hormones in all kinds of "sex-dimorphic" behavior other than sexual behavior in rodents are listed.

20. C. O. Anderson, M. X. Zarrow, and V. H. Denenberg, "Maternal Behavior in the Rabbit: Effects of Androgen Treatment during Gestation upon the Nest-Building Behaviors of the Mother and Her Offspring," *Hormones and Behaviors*, 1 (1970), 337–45, p. 338.

21. Goy and McEwen, *Sexual Differentiation*; on p. 31 we get an impression of how the male and female rat's achievements are explained: "Most sensitive to the sex difference are complex mazes with many blind alleys. Such an apparatus is really an open field with many additional walls, and, consequently it is not surprising that females make more errors since their greater level of activity and exploratory behavior translates rather directly into 'errors' in the maze."

22. John Money and Anke A. Ehrhardt, *Man and Woman, Boy and Girl: Differentiation and Dimorphism of Gender Identity from Conception to Maturity* (Baltimore: Johns Hopkins University Press, 1972).

23. You can find the criteria for the "making" of a girl or a boy in chapter 4.

24. Günther Dörner and G. Hinz, "Induction and Prevention of Male Homosexuality by Androgen," *Journal of Endocrinology*, 40 (1968), 387–88. Scientists who were interviewed considered Dörner's suggestion extreme; in this sense, Dörner should be regarded as controversial in the field of neuroendocrinology.

25. Frank Beach mentioned "a few high points" in his scientific career in his article, "Historical Origins" in 1981. He starts by mentioning his colleagues at the American Museum of Natural History and goes on to list his graduate students at Yale University and at the University of California. He received a lot of fiscal support from the National Research Council's Committee for Research on Problems on Sex. He links his history to the following disciplines: endocrinology, zoologists with special interests in behavior, neurophysiologists, neuroendocrinologists, and comparative and physiological psychologists. His own name appears in all the lists mentioned in every section devoted to a particular discipline. Frank Beach's criticism of the organization hypothesis could not be ignored. Beach died in 1988.

26. Frank A. Beach, "Hormonal Factors Controlling the Differentiation, Development and Display of Copulatory Behaviors in the Ramstergig (!) and Related Species," in E. Tobach, L. R. Aronson, and E. Shaw, eds., *The Biopsychology of Development* (New York: Academic Press, 1971), pp. 249–96.

27. For feminist authors who have formulated a critique of neuroendocrinological research on homosexuality, see Bleier, *Science and Gender,* chap. 7; Lynda Birke, *Women, Feminism and Biology* (Brighton: Harvester, 1986); and Anne Fausto-Sterling, *Myths of Gender: Biological Theories on Women and Men* (New York: Basic, 1985). See also Heino F. L. Meyer-Bahlburg, "Psychoendocrine Research on Sexual Orientation: Current Status and Future Options," *Progress in Brain Research*, 61 (1984), 375–98. For a critique on nonsexual behavior ascribed to prenatal hormonal effects, see D. M. Quadagno, R. Briscoe, and J. S. Quadagno, "Effects of Perinatal Gonadal Hormones on Selected Nonsexual Behavior Patterns: A Critical Assessment of the Nonhuman and Human Literature," *Psychological Bulletin*, 84, no. 1 (1977), 62–80.

28. This theory is just one line in the development of endocrinology, and it

emerged from many other interwoven biomedical subdisciplines. The work of Frank Lilly at the beginning of the century has been important in this instance. For an overview of the development in biomedical sciences, see Adele E. Clarke, "Embryology and the Rise of American Reproductive Sciences," in *The American Expansion of Biology,* ed. Keith Benson, Ronald Raigner, and Jane Maienschein (New Brunswick: Rutgers University Press, 1993), pp. 107–32.

29. Phoenix et al., "Organization Action," p. 370.

30. See Boers, "Wetenschap, techniek en samenleving."

31. Phoenix et al., "Organization Action," p. 381.

32. Ibid.

33. The names of the journals cited in this book give some indication of the many disciplines included. Also indicative are the variety of departments in which these authors worked, which include departments of zoology, anatomy, obstetrics, and other biomedical fields, as well as psychology and biopsychology.

34. The term "obligatory point of passage" comes from John Law, "Technology, Closure and Heterogeneous Engineering: The Case of the Portuguese Expansion," in Wiebe Bijker, Trevor Pinch, and Thomas P. Hughes, eds., *The Social Construction of Technological Systems* (Cambridge: MIT Press, 1987), pp. 111–34.

35. Money and Ehrhardt, *Man and Woman, Boy and Girl,* p. xi: "The ultimate scientific resolution of the debate will lie in surpassing the traditional, now outdated dichotomy of heredity and environment, and in properly understanding the principle of interactionism between prenatal and postnatal determinants of psychosexual differentiation, especially in connection with the principle of the critical developmental period' (for prenatal hormones to have their effects on differentiation of the brain)."

36. Money and Ehrhardt's interactionism thus had nothing to do with sociological, theoretical, and research traditions of the same name.

37. Susan Leigh Star and James R. Griesemer, "Institutional Ecology, 'Translations' and Boundary Objects: Amateurs and Professionals in Berkeley's Museum of Vertebrate Zoology, 1907–39," *Social Studies of Science,* 19 (1989), 387–420. Boundary objects are objects that are plastic enough to adapt to local needs and the constraints of the several parties employing them and yet robust enough to maintain a common identity across sites. They have different meanings in different social worlds, but their structure is common enough to more than one world to make them recognizable.

38. Richard E. Whalen, "Hormone-induced Changes in the Organization of Sexual Behavior in the Male Rat," *Journal of Comparative Physiological Psychology,* 57 (1964), 180.

39. Ibid., p. 181.

40. Nelly Oudshoorn, "Endocrinologists and the Conceptualization of Sex 1920–1940," *Journal of the History of Biology,* 23 (1990), 163–86.

41. Diana Long Hall, "Biology, Sex Hormones and Sexism in the 1920s," in Carol C. Gould and Marx Wartofsky, eds., *Women and Philosophy* (New York: Putnam, 1976), pp. 81–96.

42. Examples of titles are K. Brown-Grant, A. Munck, F. Naftolin, and M. R. Sherwood, "The Effects of the Administration of Testosterone Propionate Alone or with Phenobarbiturone and of Testosterone Metabolites to Neonatal Female Rats," *Hormones and Behavior,* 2 (1971), 173–82; and Per Södersten, "Increased Mounting Behavior in the Female Rat Following a Single Neonatal Injection of Testosterone Propionate," *Hormones and Behavior,* 4 (1973), 1–17.

The argument that the choice of the sex of experimental animals in this field is dictated by the theory becomes stronger when we consider that in the 1960s and early 1970s male rats were normally used in experiments because of problems associated with the female cycle.

43. Roger A. Gorski, "Gonadal Hormones and the Perinatal Development of Neuroendocrine Function," in L. Martini and W. F. Ganong, eds., *Frontiers in Neuroendocrinology* (New York: Oxford University Press, 1971), p. 258.

44. Ibid., pp. 252, 266.

45. Richard L. Doty, "A Cry for the Liberation of the Female Rodent: Courtship, and Copulation in Rodentia," *Psychological Bulletin,* 31 (1974), 160: "The behavior of the female has been ignored in most studies of rodent copulation. For example, during the decade from 1960 to 1969, inclusive, 68% of all studies of rat copulation published in the *Journal of Comparative and Physiological Psychology* examined only the behavior of males, and 20% only the behavior of females, and 12% the behavior of both males and females."

46. Interview with Professor Jacob J. van der Werff ten Bosch, Director, Department of Endocrinology, Erasmus University, Rotterdam, The Netherlands, December 22, 1988.

47. Some indicative titles on the relation of (prenatal) hormones and sexual orientation are: H. K. H. Brodie et al., "Plasma Testosterone Levels in Heterosexual and Homosexual Men," *New England Journal of Medicine,* 289 (1973), 1236–38; Peter Doerr et al., "Plasma Testosterone, Estradiol and Semen Analysis in Male Homosexuals," *Archives of General Psychiatry,* 29 (1973), 829–33; Peter Doerr et al., "Further Studies on Sex Hormones in Male Homosexuals," *Archives of General Psychiatry,* 33 (1976), 611–14; G. Dörner et al., "Hormonal Induction and Prevention of Female Homosexuality," *Archives of Sexual Behavior,* 4 (1979), 1–9.

48. Although this idea seems to be self-evident, it is not. There are gays whose behavior would be called feminine and lesbians (called butches) whose behavior is considered masculine. Especially in their sexual relations, however, the other sex is not involved.

49. Raymond E. Goodman, "Biology of Sexuality: Inborn Determinants of Human Sexual Response," *British Journal of Psychiatry,* 143 (1983), 216.

50. Beach, "Hormonal Factors," pp. 282, 286.

51. Ibid., pp. 286–87.

52. Ibid., p. 253.

53. Interview on April 18, 1988, with Koos Slob, Department of Endocrinology, Erasmus University, Rotterdam, The Netherlands. (Slob is studying hormonal effects on the behavior of rats and monkeys.)

54. Frank A. Beach, "Hormonal Control of Sex-Related Behavior," in Frank A. Beach, ed., *Human Sexuality in Four Perspectives* (Baltimore: Johns Hopkins University Press, 1977), p. 247.

55. The first to make this claim was Simone de Beauvoir in 1949 in *La deuxième sexe.* In the 1960s and 1970s many other feminist authors objected to the theory of biological origins of sex differences in behavior.

56. Ann Oakley, *Subject Woman* (New York: Pantheon, 1981), p. 62

57. Bleier, *Science and Gender,* esp. chap. 4; Anne Fausto-Sterling, *Myths of Gender: Biological Theories on Women and Men* (New York: Basic, 1985); Lynda Birke, *Women, Feminism and Biology: The Feminist Challenge* (Brighton: Harvester, 1986).

58. P. McDonald et al., "Failure of 5a-Dihydrotestosterone to Initiate Sexual Behavior in the Castrated Male Rat," *Nature,* 227 (1970), 964–65.

59. F. Naftolin, K. J. Ryan, and Z. Petro, "Aromatization of Androstenedione

by Limbic System Tissue from Human Fetuses," *Journal of Endocrinology,* 51 (1971), 795–96; F. Naftolin, K. J. Ryan, and Z. Petro, "Aromatization of Androstenedione by the Anterior Hypothalamus of Adult Male and Female Rats," *Endocrinology,* 90 (1972), 295–98.

60. In many articles published during the 1970s, the conversion theory is referred to as a hypothesis, and terms like "suggest" and "may be converted" are also used. This is even the case in the later work of Ryan and Naftolin. See, for example, Mary Slaughter, Richard Wilen, Kenneth J. Ryan, and Frederic Naftolin, "The Effects of Low Dose Diethylstilbestrol Administration in Neonatal Female Rats," *Journal of Steroid Biochemistry,* 8 (1977), 621–23. In 1978 the theory was referred to as a hypothesis by Richard Whalen and Anne M. Etgen, "Masculinization and Defeminization Induced in Female Hamsters by Neonatal Treatment with Estradiol Benzoate and RU–2858," *Hormones and Behavior,* 10 (1978), 170–77.

61. Richard Whalen, "Sexual Differentiation: Models, Methods and Mechanisms," in R. C. Friedman, R. M. Richart, R. L. Van de Wiele, eds., *Sex Differences in Behavior* (New York: Krüger, 1974), p. 476.

62. Roger A. Gorski, "The Neuroendocrinology of Reproduction: An Overview," *Biology of Reproduction,* 20 (1979), 113.

63. Arthur P. Arnold and Roger A. Gorski, "Gonadal Steroid Induction of Structural Sex Differences in the Central Nervous System," *Annual Review of Neuroscience,* 7 (1984), 415.

64. Bernard Shapiro, "A Paradox in Development: Masculinization of the Brain without Receptors," *Progress in Clinical Biological Research (US),* 171 (1985), 167.

65. Richard Whalen, "Multiple Actions of Steroids and Their Antagonists," *Archives of Sexual Behavior,* 13, no. 5 (1985), 498 (emphasis added).

66. S. R. Ojeda, P. S. Kalra, and S. M. McCann, "Further Studies on the Maturation of the Estrogen Negative Feedback on Gonadotropin Release in the Female Rat," *Neuroendocrinology,* 18 (1975), 242–55.

67. Klaus D. Döhler and W. Wuttke, "Changes with Age in Levels of Serum Gonadotropins, Prolactin and Gonadal Steroids in Prepubertal Male and Female Rats," *Endocrinology,* 97 (1975), 898–907.

68. John Resko, J. Ploem, and H. Stadelman, "Estrogens in Fetal and Maternal Plasma of the Rhesus Monkey," *Endocrinology,* 97 (1975), 425–30.

69. A common alternative to the term "prevent" is "to protect," which indicates a relation between a weaker and a stronger entity: the female brain, and the masculinizing effect.

70. Bruce McEwen, I. Lieberburg, C. Chaptal, and L. C. Krey, "Role of Fetoneonatal Estrogen Binding Proteins in the Association of Estrogens with Neonatal Brain Cell Nuclear Receptors," *Brain Research,* 96 (1975), 400–406.

71. Klaus D. Döhler, "Is Female Sexual Differentiation Hormone-mediated?" *Trends in Neurosciences,* 1 (1978), 138–40. Döhler raised the possibility that alpha fetoproteins are precursors of estrogen receptors.

72. R. Benno and T. Williams, "Evidence for Intracellular Localization of Alpha-foetoprotein in the Developing Rat Brain," *Brain Research,* 142 (1978), 182–86.

73. Bruce McEwen, "Gonadal Steroid Receptors in Neuroendocrine Tissues," in B. O'Malley and I. Birnbaumer, eds., *Hormone Receptors,* vol. 1, *Steroid Hormones* (New York: Academic, 1978), pp. 353–400.

74. Bruno Latour, "Give Me a Laboratory and I Will Raise the World," in

Karin Knorr and Michael Mulkay, eds., *Science Observed: Perspectives on the Social Studies of Science* (London: Sage, 1983), pp. 141–71. In this article Latour describes the evolution of the image of the anthrax disease. Pasteur's research changed perceptions of anthrax from an unpredictable affliction that recurred at random to a disease with a single cause, a microbe. "Infection" and "microbe" were new concepts with respect to anthrax and were easily introduced into society. These concepts did not exist before Pasteur's research; they were produced by science.

3. Feminism and the Biological Construction of Female and Male Behavior

1. See Susan Leigh Star, "The Sociology of the Invisible: The Primacy of Work in the Writings of Anselm Strauss," in David R. Maines, ed., *Social Organization and Social Process: Essays in Honor of Anselm Strauss* (New York: Aldine de Gruyter, 1991).

2. Increase of research in sex and gender:

Key words	Period I 1966–72	Period II 1973–77	Period III 1980–84	Rate of Increase
1. Brain growth/ development	222	410	482	2.2
2. Sex	4735	7071	6937	1.5
3. Gender	6	137	321	54
4. Combination 1 with 2 or 3	6	19	22	3.7

Note. Based on key word counts from the computer files of biomedical publications published between 1966 and 1985. Indicated is the average yearly occurrence of a key word in the three periods. Most remarkable is the increase of the key word "gender" (54x), used only in research on humans.

While the share of research concerning brain growth and development over the entire range (research including animals and humans) doubled (2.2x), research concerning brain growth or development and sex or gender practically quadrupled (3.7x). The largest increase in this type of research occurred in the period 1973–1977, after the publication of John Money and Anke Ehrhardt's *Man and Woman, Boy and Girl: Differentiation and Dimorphism of Gender Identity from Conception to Maturity* (Baltimore: Johns Hopkins University Press, 1972).

3. For example, sociobiologists adhered to genocentric (nature) theories explaining cultural phenomena and individual characteristics and produced knowledge that was incompatible with explanations by sociologists and anthropologists. See, for example, M. Sahlins, *The Use and Abuse of Biology* (London, 1977). Psychologists and biologists (experimental psychologists) argued about the "heritability" of intelligence (IQ). See, for example, P. Urbach, "Progress and Degeneration in the IQ Debate," *British Journal of the Philosophy of Science*, 25 (1974), 99–136 and 235–59.

4. See Germaine Greer, *The Female Eunuch* (London: MacGibbon and Kee, 1970).

5. These feminists are called "cultural feminists." The name "cultural feminism" was chosen by Alice Echols: "The New Feminism of Yin and Yang," in Ann Snitow, Christine Stansell, and Sharon Thompson, eds., *Powers of Desire: The*

Politics of Sexuality (New York: Monthly Review Press, 1983), pp. 439–59. Cultural feminism equates "womens's liberation with the development and preservation of a female counter culture" (p. 441). Adrienne Rich (her early work) and Mary Daly are the best known feminists in this movement.

6. Helen E. Longino, *Science as Social Knowledge: Values and Objectivity in Scientific Inquiry* (Princeton: Princeton University Press, 1990), esp. chap. 8.

7. E. Steinach, "Feminisierung von Männchen und Masculinisierung von Weibchen," *Zentralblatt für Physiology,* 27 (1913), 49.

8. The idea that homosexuality could be explained by an endocrinological theory existed as early as 1917. At that time, Frank Lillie's well-known investigations into the freemartin (a female calf that has become sterile from the hormones of a twinborn male) caught the attention of a physician working on homosexuality among psychopathic cases. In a letter, he asked Lillie about the behavior of the freemartins. Carl Moore, who worked closely with Lillie for many years, had serious doubts about attributing behavior to hormone activity. His reluctance probably indicated that behavior was not readily associated with hormone activity in the early twentieth century. See Adele Clarke, "Embryology and the Rise of American Reproductive Sciences (1910–1940)," in Keith Benson, Ronald Raigner, and Jane Maienschein, eds., *The Expansion of American Biology* (New Brunswick: Rutgers University Press, 1993), pp. 107–32.

9. C. R. Moore, "On the Physiological Properties of the Gonads as Controllers of Somatic and Psychical Characteristics," *Journal of Experimental Zoology,* 28 (1919), 137.

10. Nelly Oudshoorn, "Endocrinologists and the Conceptualization of Sex, 1920–1940," *Journal of the History of Biology,* 23, no. 2 (1990), 163–86. Nelly Oudshoorn and Marianne van den Wijngaard, "Dualism in Biology: The Case of Sex Hormones," *Women's Studies International Forum,* 14, no. 5 (1991), 459–71.

11. Phoenix et al., "Organizing Action," pp. 369–82.

12. In natural environments, both sexes of most animals exhibit both types of behavior. In experimental situations, males and females can both be tested on display of mounting as well as on lordosis.

13. As is described in the previous chapter, in the 1960s an important motivation for the research was the quest for a biological explanation for male homosexuality, traditionally considered a female-like sexuality. Based on the organization theory, scientists hypothesized that it could be caused by a lack of androgens before birth.

14. Roger A. Gorski, "Gonadal Hormones and the Perinatal Development of Neuroendocrine Function," in L. Martini and W. F. Ganong, eds., *Frontiers in Neuroendocrinology* (New York: Oxford University Press, 1971), p. 251.

15. Jaroslav Madlafousek and Zdenek Hlinak, "Sexual Behavior of the Female Laboratory Rat: Inventory, Patterning, and Measurement," *Behaviour* 63 (1977), 129–74. These Czech investigators criticized the experiments and the definitions of "stimulus females": "The control of the stimulatory situation in all the studies of male sexual behavior can be qualified as somewhat insufficient: some investigators stated only that the females used were 'receptive,' 'oestrous,' 'in heat.' Other authors, attempting to insure at least some constancy of the stimulatory situation selected females that were 'most responsive,' 'strongly receptive,' 'fully receptive,' 'exhibiting normal or typical heat behavior,' etc. The criteria used in the selection of the females lacked any elaboration of the verbally formulated intensity. The constant stimulation seems therefore to have been insufficiently controlled and not reproducible. Further, the registration of females' 'receptivity'

in the course of the experiments was altogether lacking, some investigators at best exchanging the female if her receptivity fell under the already weak criterion of selection. Insufficient and sometimes primitive control of the stimulatory field is usually in sharp contrast with the sophisticated experimental design as well as with the control of other experimental variables. This probably results from the preconception that the role of the female rat in sexual interaction is rather passive. . . . The unsubstantiated conception about the passive role of the female is apparently reinforced by the intentional preselection of vigorous males for experimental study."

16. Gorski, "Gonadal Hormones," p. 250.

17. Though the result is contrary to the expectation of the author, he did not try to explain this result, for example, by the possibility that the female might have felt more comfortable after the adaptation period.

18. Richard E. Whalen, and R. D. Nadler, "Modification of Spontaneous and Hormone Induced Sexual Behavior by Estrogen Administered to Neonatal Female Rats," *Journal of Comparative Physiological Psychology*, 60 (1965), 151.

19. Roger A. Gorski, "Modification of Ovulatory Mechanisms by Postnatal Administration of Estrogen to the Rat," *American Journal of Physiology*, 205 (1963), 842–44.

20. Frank A. Beach, "Hormonal Factors Controlling the Differentiation, Development and Display of Copulatory Behaviors in the Ramstergig (!) and Related Species," in Ethel Tobach, Lester R. Aronson and Evelyn Shaw, eds., *The Biopsychology of Development* (New York: Academic, 1971), pp. 249–96. The article concludes: "It is the purpose of this presentation to expose the weaknesses and contradictions that tend to weaken the theory that testosterone controls the organization of mechanisms in the brain which are destined to mediate copulatory behavior in adult males and females. It is suggested that at the present state of knowledge formal and quantitative statements of such relationships can better be made in terms of intervening variables based upon directly observable S-R relationships than in terms of hypothetical constructs such as imaginary mechanisms."

21. Ibid., esp. pp. 258–63.

22. Richard E. Whalen, "Hormone-induced Changes in the Organization of Sexual Behavior in the Male Rat," *Journal of Comparative Physiological Psychology*, 57 (1964), 175: "[This] led to the hypothesis that spontaneous noncopulators were males which had been adversely affected by estrogens secreted by the mother during pregnancy."

23. Beach, "Hormonal Factors."

24. From these examples of difficulties that scientists had to cope with, it seems plausible that scientists could have had reason to question the idea of the organization theory in 1960. Most results, however, were in accordance with the expectations based on the theory, thanks to the design of the experiments.

25. See Richard E. Whalen and R. W. Goy, "In Memorial, Frank A. Beach," *Hormones and Behavior*, 22 (1988), 420–21.

26. As interpreted by Juliet Mitchell, "On Freud and the Distinction between the Sexes," in Jean Strouse, ed., *Women and Analysis, Dialogues on Psychoanalytic Views of Femininity* (New York: Dell, 1974), pp. 39–50. Freud's way of thinking on sexuality was clearly still dominant in 1971. It has been acknowledged that Freud's ideas developed and functioned in a period in which thinking about masculinity and femininity can be characterized as asymmetrical and dualistic. This changed due to criticism from feminist scholars. For an overview

of feminist criticism of Freud's psychoanalysis, see Patricia Jagentowicz Mill, *Women, Nature, and Psyche* (New Haven: Yale University Press, 1987). On pages 135–46 she reviews feminist criticism of Freud as formulated by Mitchell, Irigaray, Chodorow, and others.

27. It is striking that this one-sidedness is not merely male but actually heterosexual male. An important motive among many researchers investigating hormonal effects on brain development and behavior arose from their interest in the development of male sexual behavior in order to understand male homosexual behavior, which was considered a development of female sexual behavior (see chapter 2).

28. See Gordon Bermant, "Response Latencies of Female Rats during Sexual Intercourse," *Science*, 133 (1961), 1771–73. Bermant argues that "the great majority of the studies that these and other workers have carried out focusses primary importance on the male's behavior; the female has come in for scant attention." See also John B. Calhoun, *The Ecology and Sociology of the Norway Rat* (Washington, D.C.: U.S. Government Printing Office, 1962).

29. Star, "The Sociology of the Invisible." This is what is called "articulation work."

30. In an interview with Koos Slob and Pieter van der Schoot in March 1987, each mentioned this lecture independently. It had clearly impressed them, as they were able to recall it seventeen years later.

31. B. J. Meyerson and L. H. Lindström, "Sexual Motivation in the Female Rat: A Methodological Study Applied to the Investigation of the Effects of Estradiol-benzoate," *Acta Physiologica Scandinavica*, Suppl. 389 (1973), 1–80.

32. J. Madlafousek and Z. Hlinak, "Analysis of Factors Determining the Appetitive and Aversive Phase of Sexual Behavior in the Female Rat," *Physiologica Bohemoslovenica*, 21 (1972), 416–17. By the same researchers, "The Dependence of Sexual Behavior of Inexperienced Males on the Precopulatory Behavior of Females in Albino Rat," *Physiologica Bohemoslovenica*, 21 (1972), 83–84. It is unlikely that these studies were influenced by feminist ideas. Rather, in Eastern European countries different sexual mores may have prevailed, which meant that scientists had a different perception of sexual behavior.

33. A. F. Dixon et al., "Hormonal and Other Determinants of Sexual Attractiveness and Receptivity in Rhesus and Talapoin Monkeys," IVth International Congress in Primatology 1973, vol. 2: *Primate Reproductive Behavior* (Basel: Karger, 1974), pp. 41, 42.

34. Richard L. Doty, "A Cry for the Liberation of the Female Rodent: Courtship and Copulation in Rodentia," *Psychological Bulletin*, 31 (1974), 159–73.

35. Calhoun, *Ecology and Sociology of the Norway Rat*.

36. J. Madlafousek and Z. Hlinak, "Importance of Female's Precopulatory Behaviour for the Primary Initiation of Male's Copulatory Behavior in the Laboratory Rat," *Behaviour*, 86 (1983), 237–49. The authors of this article argue that a young male rat's sexual behavior is initiated by the sexual invitation of a female rat. They associate this with the "question of the so called non-copulators," suggesting that those males simply were not "initiated": "It is an important question since the elimination of 30–40% of males from further experimentation, which is usual practice, represents great selection and weakens later generalizations."

37. Doty, "A Cry," p. 169.

38. At that time feminist thinking was mainly based on Marxist and socialist

theory. Feminists saw similarities between the liberation of women and the liberation of the suppressed working class. Feminism, therefore, was also referred to as women's liberation. These feminists pursued equal rights and equal opportunities with men.

39. Frank A. Beach, "Behavioral Endocrinology: An Emerging Discipline," *American Scientist,* 63 (1975), 179.

40. Frank A. Beach, "Sexual Attractivity, Proceptivity and Receptivity in Female Mammals," *Hormones and Behavior,* 7 (1976), 115.

41. Ibid., p. 105.

42. See Mary S. Erskine, "Solicitation Behavior in the Estrous Female Rat: A Review," *Hormones and Behavior,* 23 (1989), 473–502. The author reports that it is only in recent years that female contributions to sexual interactions have been studied. Erskine works at the Department of Biology, Boston University. See also Francien H. de Jonge, "Sexual and Aggressive Behavior in Female Rats: Psychological and Endocrine Factors" (Ph.D. thesis, University of Amsterdam, 1986); she worked at the Dutch Brain Institute. The author studied hormonal factors on sexual and aggressive behavior in female rats. She was one of the first scientists investigating aggressive behavior in females. Until then aggression was only studied in male rats, reflecting the idea that only the male is aggressive. And see D. E. Emery, "Effects of Endocrine State on Sociosexual Behavior of Female Rats Tested in a Complex Environment," *Behavioral Neuroscience,* 100 (1986), 71–78. Further, see Martha K. McClintock, J. J. Anisko, and N. J. Adler, "The Role of the Female during Copulation in Wild and Domestic Norway Rats *(Rattus norvegicus), Behaviour* (1982), 67–96. The list of female investigators might be much longer. In most laboratories where female behavior has been studied since the 1970s, a few women have contributed to the research. It is, however, difficult to tell from publications and references whether a study has been performed by a male or a female scientist. In many cases the research as well as the publication is the work of a group of people. In many cases their names are indicated with initials only; thus first names cannot give the reader an idea of the sex of the authors. Female scientists usually do not appreciate being mentioned as women; the quality of their research is more important to them.

43. The rationale behind this is that the hypothalamus is connected anatomically and functionally with the pituitary gland, which participates in the regulation of all the other endocrine glands in the body. These endocrine glands, for instance, the ovaries and the testes, in turn secrete hormones that participate in their own regulation through feedback loops acting upon the hypothalamus and the pituitary, in a manner somewhat analogous to that of a thermostat and a furnace heating system.

44. See, for example, Donna Emery and R. L. Moss, "Lesions Confined to the Ventromedial Hypothalamus Decrease the Frequency of Coital Contacts in Female Rats," *Hormones and Behavior,* 18 (1984), 313–29.

45. This did not mean that the female laboratory rat's life improved. Besides hormone injections, now she had to undergo brain surgery in the search for the part of the brain involved in coordination of sexual behavior. Marianne van den Wijngaard, "The Liberation of the Female Rodent," in Lynda Birke and Ruth Hubbard, eds., *Reinventing Biology* (Bloomington: Indiana University Press, 1995).

46. Beach, "Sexual Attractivity," p. 107.

47. In males the functions of reproduction and copulation are unified in their production of sperm. In females of many species, however, this may vary. The female rat is most likely to engage in sexual interactions during the estrous

period, during which she is fertile. In other species ovulation occurs only shortly after or during copulation. There are species in which the female permits copulation at any stage of the cycle, for example, rhesus monkeys and chimpanzees. It is remarkable that the rat model is often used to obtain understanding of human behavior, including sexual behavior.

48. Beach, "Sexual Attractivity," pp. 114, 115.

49. Ibid., p. 118.

50. Meyerson and Lindström, "Sexual Motivation."

51. John Money, "Sex Hormones and Other Variables in Human Eroticism," in W. C. Young, ed., Sex and Internal Secretions, 3rd ed. (Baltimore: Williams and Wilkins, 1961), pp. 1383–1400.

52. Beach, "Sexual Attractivity," p. 123.

53. Ibid., pp. 125, 126.

54. Ibid., p. 124.

55. B. J. Everitt, J. Herbert, and J. D. Hamer, "Sexual Receptivity of Bilaterally Adrenalectomized Female Rhesus Monkeys," Physiology of Behavior, 8 (1971), 409–15.

56. Leonore Tiefer, "The Context and Consequences of Contemporary Sex Research: A Feminist Perspective," in T. E. McGill, D. A. Dewsbury, and B. D. Sachs, eds., Sex and Behavior: Status and Prospectus (New York: Plenum, 1978), pp. 363–85.

57. Leonore Tiefer, "In memoriam, Frank A. Beach," Hormones and Behavior, 22 (1988), 441–42. This was how Beach reacted to Tiefer's presentation of her paper. Within a week he wrote her a note with an apology of sorts: "I won't be as alarmed as I was when you read it. Who knows? You might be right. I know we oldsters like to hold tight to old times and old values—often after they are no longer worth preserving. But that's why we always have a 'younger generation,' isn't it?"

58. Star, "The Sociology of the Invisible."

59. Leonore Tiefer, "Feminism and Sex Research: Ten Years' Reminiscences and Appraisal," in Joan C. Chrisler and Doris Howard, eds., New Directions in Feminist Psychology (New York: Springer, 1992).

60. In a letter written on March 5, 1990, in which she answered my question about her perceptions of developments in the field.

61. Beach, "Sexual Attractivity," p. 131.

62. Günther Dörner and G. Hinz, "Induction and Prevention of Male Homosexuality by Androgen," Journal of Endocrinology, 40 (1968), 387–88.

63. Money and Ehrhardt, Man and Woman, Boy and Girl.

64. John Money, Love and Love Sickness: The Science of Sex, Gender Difference, and Pair-bonding (Baltimore: Johns Hopkins University, 1980). Money calls the behavior studied with regard to the prenatal effects of androgens "sex-shared/threshold-dimorphic behavior." This type of behavior consists of nine variables, among which are sexual behavior and the expenditure of energy in sport and games.

65. An example is the publication by Irvin Yalom, Richard Green, and Norman Fisk, "Prenatal Exposure to Female Hormones: Effect on Psychosexual Development in Boys," Archives of General Psychiatry, 28 (1973), 554–62. To give the reader an idea of what was measured and what was regarded as "masculine," I will quote part of the description of the structured interviews:

aggressivity ranking: Presence of any aggressive activities, for example, hunting, fighting, and rough-and-tumble elements; preferred content of television, books, and movies (presence of particularly aggressive themes—war, fighting); future goals (presence of particularly aggressive careers (e.g., FBI agent, race car driver); military service (either an eagerness to join the military or a firm stand on a refusal to enter the military were given high aggressive rating); number and severity of injuries; frankly aggressive behavior (level in physical power hierarchy in the class, disciplinary problems); and selection of aggressive heroes.

masculine interest: Tinkering with automobile engines was given a high masculine rating, while drawing, writing, listening to records, and photography tended to be given a lower masculine interest; sports (here the emphasis is on masculine interest rather than sheer aggressivity; e.g., weight lifting would be given a high masculine interest rating but not a high aggressivity rating), hobbies, and academic subjects. (Most masculine would be mathematics, science, physical education, mechanical drawing; the least masculine would be art, English, languages, and music.) Fantasied and realistic goals, adventuresome nature, competitiveness, and level of aspiration (high masculine ratings included astronaut, the first man to dive 300 feet under water, head of the FBI, gym teacher, motorcycle driver; whereas least masculine would be music composer, actor). Heroes (most masculine would be such people as John Wayne and Marlon Brando, some of the least masculine would be Louis Pasteur, the pope, and Walt Whitman).

heterosexual development: Number of girlfriends, amount of social and physical contact with girls, contact with pornography, frequency of masturbation and fantasy content with masturbation, homosexual play, and other factors.

66. Eleanor Maccoby and Carol Jacklin, *The Psychology of Sex Differences* (Stanford: Stanford University Press, 1974), p. 2.

67. Ibid., p. 2.

68. Ibid., p. 7.

69. Ibid., pp. 12, 13.

70. For a methodological discussion about the possibility of the role of biology in the differences found by Maccoby and Jacklin, see Ruth Bleier, *Science and Gender: A Critique of Biology and Its Theories on Women* (New York: Pergamon, 1984), esp. chap. 4: "Hormones, the Brain and Sex Differences." Bleier argues that it is impossible to analyze the biological "fundamentals" of human behavior "uncontaminated" by culture. See also Anne Fausto-Sterling, *Myths of Gender: Biological Theories on Women and Men* (New York: Basic, 1988). Fausto-Sterling explores the possibility that the statistics in these "statistically significant" differences are intellectually meaningless. According to her, even if they are not meaningless, the differences are too small to account for the small number of women in, for example, engineering jobs, for which these differences in skills are often used as an argument. Moreover she noted that the experimenters were mostly men, which probably affected the differences in results between females and males.

71. Maccoby and Jacklin, *Psychology of Sex Differences,* p. 360.

72. Ibid., p. 361.

73. See Norman Geschwind and Albert Galaburda, "Cerebral Lateralization," *Archives of Neurology,* 42 (1985), 428–59. These scientists ascribe the higher occurrence in men of left-handedness, susceptibility to allergies, learning disabilities, and superior mathematical performance to prenatal hormone exposure of the brain. They guessed that fetal testosterone might influence the degree of hemispheric functional asymmetry. See also Camilla Benbow and Julian Stanley, "Sex Differences in Mathematical Ability: Fact or Artefact?" *Science,* 210 (1980), 1262–64. These scientists suggested that the differences in spatial tasks and superior male mathematical ability originated in a genetic difference.

74. For an overview of the research and the variables involved, see a report of

a conference entitled "Biological Foundations of Cerebral Dominance," April 4–6, 1983, in Boston, under the joint sponsorship of the Harvard Department of Neurology and the Institute for Child Development Research. The purpose of the meeting was a unified presentation of the developed biological approaches to the study of cerebral laterality. See also Norman Geschwind, "Biological Foundations of Cerebral Dominance," *Trends in Neurosciences,* 6, no. 9 (1983), 354–56.

75. David M. Quadagno, Robert Briscoe, and Jill S. Quadagno, "Effect of Perinatal Gonadal Hormones on Selected Nonsexual Behavior Patterns: A Critical Assessment of the Nonhuman and Human Literature," *Psychological Bulletin,* 84 (1977), 62–80. The first two authors had published before in this field of research; they worked at the Department of Physiology and Cell Biology. Jill Quadagno worked in the Sociology Department. Although the content of the article makes this combination of researchers plausible, it is remarkable that two researchers from the biomedical sciences published the article with a sociologist. Jill Quadagno was inspired by feminist ideas concerning environmental explanations for sex differences, though this is not explicitly mentioned in the article. Contrary to the practice in psychological publications, feminist involvement is usually not mentioned as a motivation for research in the biomedical sciences.

76. Ibid., p. 69.

77. Froukje M. E. Slijper, "Androgens and Gender Role Behavior in Girls with Congenital Adrenal Hyperplasia (CAH)," *Progress in Brain Research,* 61 (1984), 421. In 1983 Slijper published a thesis on how being ill affected the display of "tomboy" behavior: *Gender Role Behavior in Girls with Congenital Adrenal Hyperplasia* (Ph.D. thesis, Department of Child Psychiatry, Erasmus University, Rotterdam).

78. Celia Moore, "Maternal Behavior of Rats Is Affected by Hormonal Condition of Pups," *Journal of Comparative and Physiological Psychology,* 96, no. 1 (1982), 123–29.

79. Celia Moore, "Maternal Contributions to the Development of Masculine Sexual Behavior in Laboratory Rats," *Developmental Psychobiology,* 17 (1984), 347–56; Celia Moore, "Another Psychobiological View of Sexual Differentiation," *Developmental Review,* 5 (1985), 18–55.

80. Anke A. Ehrhardt and Heino F. L. Meyer-Bahlburg, "Effects of Prenatal Sex Hormones on Gender-related Behavior," *Science,* 211 (1981), 1312–18.

81. John Money and A. J. Russo, "Homosexual Outcome of Discordant Gender Identity/Role in Childhood: Longitudinal Follow-up," *Journal of Pediatric Psychology,* 4 (1979), 29–41.

82. F. Naftolin, "Understanding the Bases of Sex Differences," *Science,* 211 (1981), 1264.

83. Since the 1940s physicians had prescribed for women different types of estrogens and progestagens during gestation. The most frequently used hormone was diethyl stilbestrol (DES). They expected that these hormones could prevent premature birth in cases of diabetes or other illnesses that were thought to be linked to deficiencies of hormone production. Supplementation seemed to be the logical treatment and was strongly advised by the pharmaceutical industry. Later, prenatal exposure to DES was found to be associated with a highly increased risk of the development of a rare form of cancer in the daughters. Also, menstrual irregularities and pregnancy problems occurred. DES sons showed a variety of genito-urinary disorders.

84. Scientists also regarded it as advantageous that the DES children's hormonal status was more equivalent to that of experimental animals: the source of

their abnormal hormonal environment was exogenous—whereas the source of the abnormal hormones in the intersexes was endogenous, resulting from abnormalities in genes, enzymes, or adrenals.

85. See, for example, P. Södersten and J. A. Gustafsson, "A Way in Which Estradiol Might Play a Role in the Sexual Behavior of Male Rats," *Hormones and Behavior,* 14 (1980), 271–74.

86. Melissa Hines, "Prenatal Gonadal Hormones and Sex Differences in Human Behavior," *Psychological Bulletin,* 92 (1982), 76.

87. Anke A. Ehrhardt, "Gender Differences: A Biosocial Perspective," in Richard A. Dienstbier and Theo B. Sonderegger, eds., *Current Theory and Research in Motivation,* vol. 32 (Lincoln: University of Nebraska Press, 1985), pp. 37–59.

88. June M. Reinisch, "Effects of Prenatal Hormone Exposure on Physical and Psychological Development in Humans and Animals: With a Note on the State of the Field," in Edward J. Sachar, ed., *Hormones, Behavior, and Psychopathology* (New York: Raven, 1976), pp. 70–94.

89. Ehrhardt, "Gender Differences," p. 48.

90. Ibid., p. 49.

91. Consider, for example, the percentage of length of discussion in relation to total text (excluding references) in the following papers published by Anke Ehrhardt with other scientists:

I. Ehrhardt, Anke A., G. C. Grisanti, and H. F. L. Meyer-Bahlburg, "Prenatal Exposure to Medroxyprogesterone Acetate (MPA) in Girls," *Psychoneuroendocrinology,* 2 (1977), 391–98.

II. Ehrhardt, Anke A., S. E. Ince, and H. F. L. Meyer-Bahlburg, "Career Aspiration and Gender Role Development in Young Girls," *Archives of Sexual Behavior,* 10, no. 3 (1981), 281–99.

III. Heino F. L. Meyer-Bahlburg, A. A. Ehrhardt, L. R. Rosen, J. F. Feldman, N. P. Veridiano, I. Zimmerman, and B. S. McEwen, "Psychosexual Milestones in Women Prenatally Exposed to Diethylbestrol," *Hormones and Behavior,* 18 (1984), 359–66.

IV. Ehrhardt, Anke A., H. F. L. Meyer-Bahlburg, L. R. Rosen, J. F. Feldman, N. P. Veridiano, I. Zimmerman, and B. S. McEwen, "Sexual Orientation after Prenatal Exposure to Exogenous Estrogen," *Archives of Sexual Behavior,* 14, no. 1 (1985), 57–75:

	I (1977)	II (1981)	III (1984)	IV (1985)
discussion	1.5	3	2	5
text	6	13.5	3.5	11
amount of discussion	25%	22%	56%*	46%

*This discussion includes a table.

92. Pieter van der Schoot and A. Kooy, "Current Topics in the Study of Sexual Behavior in Rats," in J. M. A. Sitsen, ed., *Handbook of Sexology,* vol. 6: *The Pharmacology and Endocrinology of Sexual Function* (Amsterdam: Elsevier, 1988), pp. 145–92. As summarized by the authors in defending the validity of the theory: Some believe "that differences in sexual behaviour can be wholly explained by the different gonadal hormonal milieu in adulthood together with the different sexual experiences animals have due to different external genital anatomy" (p. 173).

93. For an overview of the discussion, see Mary Vetterling-Braggin, ed.,

"Femininity," "Masculinity" and "Androgyny": A Modern Philosophical Discussion (Totowa, N.J.: Littlefield Adams, 1982). The authors deal with the central question of whether the "masculine" is male-linked and the "feminine" female-linked with respect both to psychological characteristics and to social and labor roles. Various notions of sex and gender in the literature are discussed and tested, and the methodological difficulties in confirming a presupposed sex-gender link are examined. A substantial portion of the book is devoted to the pros and cons of "androgyny."

94. Sandra L. Bem, "The Measurement of Psychological Androgyny," *Journal of Consulting and Clinical Psychology*, 42 (1972), 155–62; Anne Constantinople, "Masculinity-Femininity: An Exception to a Famous Dictum?" *Psychological Bulletin*, 80, no. 5 (1973), 389–407. See also Janet T. Spence, Robert Helmreich, and Joy Stapp, "Ratings of Self and Peers on Sex Role Attributes and Their Relation to Self-Esteem and Conceptions of Masculinity and Femininity," *Journal of Personality and Social Psychology*, 32, no. 1 (1975), 29–39.

95. In this period it was recognized that in natural situations both male and female rats have the ability to display types of sexual behavior that in laboratory experiments were defined as masculine or feminine sexual behavior. Nanne van der Poll, *Bisexual Behavior in the Male and Female Rat* (Ph.D. thesis, University of Amsterdam, 1974). He argued that the suggestion that sexual behavior was bipolar (male or female), which was accepted at that time, was misleading.

96. In an interview at a conference of the International Academy of Sex Research in Prague on July 9, 1992, Whalen told me he was inspired by Bem's work. He did not answer my question about why he did not refer to her work in his article.

97. Richard Whalen, "Sexual Differentiation: Models, Methods and Mechanisms," in R. C. Friedman, R. M. Richart, and R. L. Van de Wiele, eds., *Sex Differences in Behavior* (New York: Krüger, 1974), pp. 467–81.

98. Reinisch, "Effects of Prenatal Hormone Exposure," pp. 70–94.

99. Ibid., p. 84.

100. June M. Reinisch and W. G. Karow, "Prenatal Exposure to Synthetic Progestins and Estrogens: Effects on Human Development," *Archives of Sexual Behavior*, 6 (1977), 257–88.

101. Synthetic progestins were originally considered as replacements for "female" pregnancy hormones. In the research on their effects on behavior it turned out that "they could not be equated as a group with progesterone, because some are inherently estrogenic, some slightly androgenic, and some pure progestational. In addition, progestins may vary in potency"; L. S. Goodman and A. Gilman, *The Pharmacological Basis of Therapeutics*, 5th ed. (New York: Macmillan, 1975), p. 1439.

102. Reinisch, "Effects of Prenatal Hormone Exposure," p. 81.

103. June M. Reinisch, "Prenatal Exposure of Human Foetuses to Synthetic Progestin and Oestrogen Affects Personality," *Nature*, 266 (1977), 561–62. The factor "corteric" is lacking in these results. This publication appeared in the references of Reinisch's article in *Hormones and Behavior*, but not vice versa.

104. Melissa Hines, "Prenatal Diethylstilbestrol (DES) Exposure, Human Sexually Dimorphic Behavior and Cerebral Lateralization" (Ph.D. dissertation, University of California, Los Angeles, 1981), *Dissertation Abstracts International*, 42 (1981), 423B.

105. Melissa Hines, "Prenatal Gonadal Hormones and Sex Differences in Human Behavior," *Psychological Bulletin*, 92, no. 1 (1982), 69.

106. June M. Reinisch, "Prenatal Exposure to Synthetic Progestins Increases Potential for Aggression in Humans," *Science,* 211 (1981), 1171–73.

107. For a critical discussion of research methodology on DES daughters and sons and Reinisch's contributions, see Anne Fausto-Sterling, *Myths of Gender: Biological Theories on Women and Men* (New York: Basic, 1988), esp. pp. 138–42.

108. See Oudshoorn and van den Wijngaard, "Dualism in Biology," pp. 459–71. This article describes how during the twentieth century androgens and estrogens were believed to function as messengers for masculinity and femininity, respectively.

109. See Judith Walzer Leavitt and Linda Gordon, "A Decade of Feminist Critiques in the Natural Sciences: An Address by Ruth Bleier," *Signs: Journal of Women in Culture and Society,* 14, no. 1 (1988), 182–96.

110. See, for example, Christine de Lacoste-Utamsing and Ralph Holloway, "Sexual Dimorphism in the Human Corpus Callosum," *Science,* 216 (1982), 1431–32; Dick Swaab and E. Fliers, "A Sexually Dimorphic Nucleus in the Human Brain," *Science,* 228 (1985), 1112–16.

111. Many articles in newspapers and journals on the subject of differences in male and female brains were published. Several books were devoted to the subject, for example, John Durden-Smith and Diana De Simone, *Sex and the Brain* (London: Pan, 1983); Anne Moir and David Jessel, *BrainSex: The REAL Difference between MEN and WOMEN* (London: Michael Joseph, 1989).

112. Moir and Jessel, *BrainSex.*

113. Piet Vroon, "Seksen," in the Dutch newspaper *De Volkskrant* on August 18, 1990. He publicly revised his opinion referring to my thesis (which forms the basis for this book) in an interview in the Dutch feminist magazine *Opzij* of March 1994. Piet Vroon is a well-known publicist and psychologist in The Netherlands.

114. See also Anne Fausto-Sterling, "Life in the XY Corral," *Women's Studies International Forum,* 12, no. 3 (1989), 319–31; and Anne Fausto-Sterling, "Society Writes Biology, Biology Constructs Gender," *Daedalus* 116 (1987), 61–76. In these papers she examines how and to what degree sociopolitical categories of race, gender, and class have left their mark on the field of developmental biology and genetics. Also in these fields of biology, femaleness is associated with absence or passivity and maleness with presence and activity.

115. Thomas Laqueur, *Making Sex: Body and Gender from the Greeks to Freud* (Cambridge: Harvard University Press, 1990).

116. Dorothy Price, "Feedback Control of Gonadal and Hypophyseal Hormones: Evolution of the Concept," in Joseph Meites, Bernal T. Donovan, Samuel M. McCann, eds., *Pioneers in Neuroendocrinology* (New York: Plenum, 1975), pp. 219–39. Dorothy Price was an eminent scientist and in May 1930 she developed the understanding of the feedback mechanism regulating secretion of hypothalamic and gonadal hormones. The mechanism is called the Moore-Price feedback mechanism. Moore was her supervisor; he was inspired by her and claimed that he developed the theory. Price writes on page 221: "Moore was a male chauvinist, and women (with the possible exception of a few including me on some occasions) were not really to be considered scientifically equal to men. I think he did not realize the depth of his prejudice. . . . I was quite willing to be 'appropriated'. . . . I chose to disregard it then as much I could and I accept male chauvinism now with resignation and a certain measure of amusement . . . . Most men really can't help it, Dorothy; it's all that terrible male hormone." And

on page 235 she writes: "Still I am glad that in May 1930 I did not know what was going on in the minds of so many. It would have spoiled part of the fun."

117. Helen E. Longino, *Science as Social Knowledge: Values and Objectivity in Scientific Inquiry* (Princeton: Princeton University Press, 1990), p. 171.

4. The Construction of Women and Men in Medical Practice

1. The term "obligatory point of passage" comes from John Law, "Technology, Closure and Heterogeneous Engineering: The Case of the Portuguese Expansion," in Wiebe Bijker, Trevor Pinch, and Thomas P. Hughes, eds., *The Social Construction of Technological Systems* (Cambridge: MIT Press, 1987), pp. 111–34.

2. Hermaphrodites are animals with male as well as female genital organs and are capable of self-fertilization. This feature is common to invertebrates. While it does not occur in human beings, pseudohermaphroditism does; that is to say, there are cases where the outer characteristics and build of the genital organs are between the sexes. Pseudohermaphrodites are, therefore, also referred to as intersex.

3. John Money, Joan G. Hampson, and John L. Hampson, "An Examination of Some Basic Sexual Concepts: The Evidence of Human Hermaphroditism," *Bulletin Johns Hopkins Hospital*, 97 (1955), 301–19. The authors discussed data from seventy-six children reared as either boys or girls, often in contradiction to external genitalia, chromosomes, or hormonal activity. They note (p. 308): "From the sum total of hermaphrodic evidence, the conclusion that emerges is that sexual behavior and orientation as male or female does not have an innate, instinctive basis. . . . In place of a theory of instinctive masculinity or femininity which is innate, the evidence . . . lends support to a conception that, psychologically, sexuality is undifferentiated at birth and that it becomes differentiated as masculine or feminine in the course of various experiences of growing up."

4. The frequencies of counseling vary depending on the hospital's facilities. Some patients see the endocrinologist once a year, others see a psychiatrist of a special gender team weekly (e.g., at Erasmus University, Rotterdam, The Netherlands).

5. S. Kessler and W. McKenna, "Toward a Theory of Gender," in *Gender, an Ethnomethodological Approach* (New York: Wiley, 1978).

6. Barbara Fried, "What Is a Woman?" in Ruth Hubbard, Mary Sue Henifin, and Barbara Fried, *Women Look at Biology Looking at Women* (Cambridge: Schenkman, 1978).

7. Stefan Hirschauer, "The Manufacture of Bodies in Surgery," *Social Studies of Science*, 21 (1991), 279–319.

8. To answer these questions, I analyzed fifty-nine texts published between 1972 and 1989 in three well-read medical journals: *The Lancet, The New England Journal of Medicine*, and the *Nederlands Tijdschrift voor Geneeskunde* (Dutch Journal of Medicine).

9. R. Whitley, "The Establishment and Structure of the Sciences as Reputational Organizations," in N. Elias, H. Maihns, and R. Whitley, eds., *Scientific Establishments and Hierarchies, Sociology of the Sciences Yearbook* (Dordrecht: Reidel, 1982).

10. Susan L. Star, "Scientific Work and Uncertainty," *Social Studies of Science*,

15 (1985), 391–427; idem, "Simplification in Scientific Work: An Example from Neuro-endocrine Research," *Social Studies of Science,* 13 (1983), 205–208.

11. *Oosthoek Encyclopedie,* 1980 edition.

12. G. H. Herdt and J. Davidson, "The Sambia 'Turnim-man': Socio-cultural and Clinical Aspects of Gender Formation in Male Pseudohermaphrodites with 5 Alpha Reductase Deficiency in Papua New Guinea," *Archives of Sexual Behavior,* 17, no. 1 (1988), 33. Other examples of the occurrence of a third sex appear among the Ngadju of Borneo and in southern Sulawesi. These people are called *basir* and *bissu,* respectively.

13. Kessler and McKenna, "Toward a Theory of Gender." This provocative study focuses on challenges to common ideas about gender: the phenomenon of transsexualism, some ideas that children have about gender, and the treatment of gender in other cultures.

14. Michel Foucault brought the existence and the experiences of a pseudohermaphrodite to the attention of a larger public by publishing *Herculine Barbin, dite Alexina B. presenté par Michel Foucault* (Paris: Gallimard, 1978). Foucault suggests that the medical term "pseudo" in this case means that there is an underlying real male or female to be discovered by medical examination (p. 190).

15. Julia Epstein, "Either/Or–Neither/Both: Sexual Ambiguity and the Ideology of Gender," *Genders,* 7 (1990), 99–142; idem, *Altered Conditions: Disease, Medicine and Storytelling* (New York: Routledge, 1995).

16. Randolph Trumbach, "London Sodomites: Homosexual Behavior and Western Culture in the Eighteenth Century," *Journal of Social History,* 11 (1977), 1–33. Trumbach associates the impossibility of the existence of a third sex in European cultures with their opposition to all forms of homosexuality.

17. Epstein, "Either/Or–Neither/Both"; Anne Fausto-Sterling, "The Five Sexes: Why Male and Female Are Not Enough," *The Sciences* (March-April 1993), 20–24. The author provides strong arguments for social acceptance of pseudohermaphrodites by distinguishing five sexes instead of two. The recognition of five sexes can open opportunities for intersex people to live a more human life than with a medical history of surgery and hormone treatments. Scarring often leads to loss of orgasm and patients with these operations are very aware of their physical differences.

18. A. Jost, "Hormonal Influences in the Development of the Fetus," *Cold Spring Harbor Symposium on Quantitative Biology,* 19 (1954), 3–9.

19. John Money, *Love and Love Sickness: The Science of Sex, Gender Difference and Pair-Bonding* (Baltimore: Johns Hopkins University Press, 1980), p. 5: "The principle involved, nicknamed the Adam Principle, is the same as governs the differentiation of the genital anatomy, namely, that to differentiate a male something must be added." In relation to the above, another passage is quite remarkable: M. Mellcow Meyer, "Tumors of Dysgenetic Gonads in Intersexes: Case Reports and Discussion Regarding Their Place in Gonadal Oncology," *Bulletin of the New York Academy of Medicine,* 42, no. 3 (1966): "The 'battle of the sexes' begins early in intrauterine life. Gestation takes place in a maternal estrogenic environment. Thus it becomes necessary, in dealing with male embryos, to have some factors to counteract this influence, else all individuals, irrespective of genotype, would be born as female phenotypes."

20. John Money and Anke A. Ehrhardt, *Man and Woman, Boy and Girl: Differentiation and Dimorphism of Gender Identity from Conception to Maturity* (Baltimore: Johns Hopkins University Press, 1972).

21. D. Federman, "Psychosexual Adjustment in Congenital Adrenal Hyperplasia," *New England Journal of Medicine,* 316 (1987), 210.

22. Fausto-Sterling, "The Five Sexes," pp. 20–24.

23. E. Braunwald, ed., *Harrison's Principles of Internal Medicine,* 11th ed. (New York: McGraw-Hill, 1987).

24. Personal communication with Fausto-Sterling. Soon she will publish *Building Bodies: Biology and the Social Construction of Sexuality.*

25. I. Huyts, *Niet Vrouw, Niet Man: Beelden van vrouwelijkheid en mannelijkheid in biologie en geneeskunde.* "Verslag van een doktoraal onderzoek. Vrouwenstudies Biologie," University of Amsterdam, 1988.

26. See G. Richardson, "Case 8–1977," *New England Journal of Medicine,* 296 (1977), 439: "She had always been tall and of exceptional physical strength." See also J. Griffin and J. Wilson, "The Syndromes of Androgen Resistance," *New England Journal of Medicine,* 302 (1980), 201: "The general habitus and the distribution of body fat are female in character."

27. In the 1950s, scientists advised doctors to postpone surgical correction until after puberty since changes in the sex of a child with ambiguous genitals could sometimes occur later: "It is best if the sex is doubtful at birth to register and rear the child as a male, first, because most pseudo-hermaphrodites are males, and secondly because a male in a girls' school can do a lot of harm before his true sex is discovered. It is best to delay decision as to the true sex until puberty when the secondary sex characters declare themselves"; in F. Browne, *Postgraduate Obstetrics and Gynecology* (London: Butterworths, 1950).

28. A. Vos, "Pseudohermafroditisme," *Nederlands Tydschrift voor Geneeskunde,* 119 (1975), 1923: "In therapy, the anatomical deviation is paramount: when it is impossible to construct a functioning phallus, it is preferable to consider the individual a woman" (translation M.v.d.W.).

29. Federman, "Psychosexual Adjustment," p. 210: "the heterosexual adjustment of adult patients with congenital adrenal hyperplasia (form of pseudohermaphroditism) correlates with the adequacy of the introitus. . . ."

30. J. Dewhurst and R. Gordon, "Fertility Following Change of Sex: A Follow Up," *Lancet* (1984), ii, 1461.

31. J. Aiman, J. Griffin, J. Gazak, J. Wilson, and P. MacDonald, "Androgen Insensitivity as a Cause of Infertility in Otherwise Normal Men," *New England Journal of Medicine,* 300 (1979), 223.

32. J. van Dijk, "Een geval van interseksualiteit," *Nederlands Tydschrift voor Geneeskunde,* 119 (1975), 691.

33. For example, J. Pronk, ed., *Medische genetica* (Utrecht: Bunge, 1984); J. Forfar and G. Arneil, eds., *Textbook of Paediatrics,* 3rd ed. (Edinburgh: Churchill Livingstone, 1984); G. Kloosterman, ed., *De voortplanting van de mens, leerboek voor obstetrie en gynaecologie,* 7th ed. (Weesp: Centen, 1985); H. Kaplan and B. Sadock, eds., *Modern Synopsis of Comprehensive Textbook of Psychiatry,* 4th ed. (Baltimore: Williams & Wilkins, 1985); J. Wilson and D. Foster, eds., *Williams Textbook of Endocrinology,* 7th ed. (Philadelphia: Saunders, 1985); E. Braunwald, ed., *Harrison's Principles of Internal Medicine,* 11th ed. (New York: McGraw-Hill, 1987); V. Tindall, *Jeffcoate's Principles of Gynecology,* 5th ed. (London: Butterworth, 1987).

34. Money and Ehrhardt, *Man and Woman, Boy and Girl.*

35. The first person who saw prenatal hormones as the cause for homosexuality was Günther Dörner. See G. Dörner and G. Hinz, "Induction and Prevention of Male Homosexuality by Androgen," *Journal of Endocrinology,* 40 (1968), 387–88.

36. Money, *Love and Love Sickness*. Money calls the behavior studied with regard to the prenatal effects of androgens "sex-shared/threshold-dimorphic behavior." This type of behavior consists of nine variables, including sexual behavior and the expenditure of energy in sport and games.

37. J. Imperato-McGinley, R. Peterson, T. Gautier, and E. Sturla, "Androgens and the Evolution of Male Gender Identity among Male Pseudohermaphrodites with 5 Alpha-reductase Deficiency," *New England Journal of Medicine*, 300 (1979), 1233–37. The following provides more information about the image of masculinity held by the authors: "The manifestations of male sexual behavior were evaluated according to four patterns of sexual behavior differentiation described by Diamond (1977): sexual gender identity, sexual patterns (sex-related behavior, which for men includes direct aggressiveness, assertiveness, large motor activity and occupation), sexual object of choice (the sex of the person chosen as an erotically interesting partner) and sexual mechanisms (the features of sexual expression over which an individual has little control, which for men include the ability to obtain and maintain an erection and to achieve orgasm)" (p. 1234).

38. Ibid.

39. J. Griffin and J. Wilson, "The Syndromes of Androgen Resistance," *New England Journal of Medicine*, 302 (1980), 202.

40. J. Ladee-Levy, F. Slijper, S. Drop, J. Molenaar, R. Scholtmeyer, "Psychosociale gevolgen van ontwikkelingsstoornissen van de geslachtsorganen," *Nederlands Tydschrift voor Geneeskunde*, 130 (1986), 1556–59. These authors give a definition of "tomboy" behavior in girls: "At primary school age, all five exhibited clear "tomboy" behavior, consisting of rough and tumble play, a preference for boys' toys (trains, etc.) and boys' play (robbers, soldiers, etc.), boys' clothes and a dislike of girlish frills" (trans. M.v.d.W.), p. 1557.

41. Dewhurst and Gordon, "Fertility Following Change of Sex," p. 1461.

42. N. Oudshoorn and M. A. van den Wijngaard, "Dualism in Biology: The Case of Sex-hormones," *Women's Studies International Forum*, 14, no. 5 (1991), 459–71.

43. See Star, "Scientific Work and Uncertainty."

44. The following passage provides an example: "In normal males the development of the female type of breasts at puberty is thought to be prevented by an androgenic influence on the breast *anlage* during fetal life, and, of course, patients with insensitivity to testosterone lack this influence. Finally, the central nervous system is probably also androgen-insensitive in these patients since they have a characteristically female psychosexual orientation. Androgens increase libido in females, and insensitivity to them in this patient is consistent with the remark in the case record that her libido was never very strong" (*Anlage* is German for "predisposition"); G. Richardson, "Case 8–1977," *New England Journal of Medicine*, 296 (1977), 441. It is remarkable that this passage attributes the female libido to androgens, a fact which is disputed. Many research results attribute an increase in the libido to a high concentration of estrogens and progesterone, which reach their highest levels around ovulation. During this period, the chance of fertilization is at its peak. It seems as if these publications view the increase in the libido as a function of reproduction. In the passage above, the libido is obviously regarded as sexual or masculine and, therefore, as a function of androgens.

45. R. Williams, *Textbook of Endocrinology*, 6th ed. (Philadelphia: Saunders, 1985).

46. Nevertheless, discussion of whether and to what extent hormones can

determine human behavior before birth did take place in the journals. The authors of the articles held different opinions.

47. Whitley, "The Establishment and Structure."

48. Not all doctors share these ideas. In this area, it involves publication by authors who publish in renowned journals. The status of the journals and the nature of the subject may have contributed to the interpretation of the images of femininity and masculinity. A selection of those who have published on this subject in these journals may have taken place. A doctor of established reputation was probably more likely to have his work published in such a journal than less-experienced colleagues. And this area involves a deviation about which it is also conceivable that senior physicians will publish more readily than junior doctors.

49. Anke A. Ehrhardt, Heino F. L. Meyer-Bahlburg, Laura R. Rosen, Judith F. Feldman, Norma P. Veridiano, I. Zimmerman, and Bruce S. McEwen, "Sexual Orientation after Prenatal Exposure to Exogenous Estrogen," *Archives of Sexual Behavior,* 14 (1985), 57–76. They conclude (p. 72): "Findings on sexual orientation in individuals with hormonal abnormalities or particular hormonal treatment regimens during fetal life may not have any bearing on the etiology in bisexual or homosexual individuals without such medical histories. Therefore, any conclusions from the data on the specific samples of our study to the development of sexual orientation in general seem unwarranted at this time."

50. Anonymous, "Once a Dark Secret," *British Medical Journal,* 305 (February 19, 1994), 542; Anonymous, "Be Open and Honest with Sufferers," *British Medical Journal,* 306 (April 16, 1994), 1041–42. This article includes three addresses of support groups in England. The address of the Intersex Society of North America is: P.O. Box 31791, San Francisco, CA 94131.

51. A. P. van Seters and A. K. Slob, "Mutually Gratifying Heterosexual Relationship with Micropenis of Husband," *Journal of Sex and Marital Therapy,* 14 (1988), 97–104.

5. Reinventing the Sexes

1. See, for example, Robert Trivers, "Parental Investment and Sexual Selection," in *Sexual Selection and the Descent of Man,* B. Campbell, ed. (Chicago: Aldine, 1972); E. O. Wilson, *Sociobiology: The New Synthesis* (Cambridge: Belknap, 1975); idem, *On Human Nature* (New York: Bantam, 1979); Richard Dawkins, *The Selfish Gene* (Oxford: Oxford University Press, 1976).

2. A selective list of the many journals founded during the 1970s and publishing research on biological factors affecting behavior includes *Behavioral Biology: An Interdisciplinary Journal* (U.S., 1972); *Behavioral and Neural Biology: An Interdisciplinary Journal* (U.S., 1979); *Behavioral and Brain Sciences* (U.K., 1978); *Behavioral Ecology and Sociobiology* (Federal Republic of Germany, 1976); *Behavioral Brain Research: An International Journal* (The Netherlands, 1980).

3. Thomas Laqueur, *Making Sex: Body and Gender from the Greeks to Freud* (Cambridge: Harvard University Press, 1990).

4. Before 1959 endocrinologists investigated the effects of prenatal hormones on the later function of the hypothalamus. They found that the absence of androgens made the later release of the hypothalamus cyclical (or female), while their presence made this release acyclical (or male). Embryologists suggested that the presence of androgens resulted in male genital development, whereas their absence resulted in female genital development.

5. The presence or absence of androgens in sex determination as well as with regard to behavioral development is still very strong. If you read modern textbooks or the current literature on sex, you will see it repeated many times.

6. For a critical discussion of Money and Ehrhardt's work, see Ruth Bleier, *Science and Gender: A Critique of Biology and Its Theories on Women* (New York: Pergamon, 1984), esp. chap. 4; Anne Fausto-Sterling, *Myths of Gender: Biological Theories on Women and Men* (New York: Basic, 1988); Lynda Birke, *Women, Feminism and Biology: The Feminist Challenge* (Brighton: Harvester, 1986).

7. For example, D. F. Swaab and M. A. Hofman, "Sexual Differentiation of the Human Brain: A Historical Perspective," *Progress in Brain Research*, 61 (1984), 361–75. These authors explicitly oppose feminist author Greer by providing accounts of all sorts of differences in human brains, including sex differences in microscopic structures in the brain and differing brain weights and sizes, those of women being smaller. They argue (p. 367) that "it seems plausible to suppose that intelligence is determined in part by the amount of brain tissue in excess of that required for receiving sensory information and controlling muscle movements."

8. Richard Whalen, "Multiple Actions of Steroids and Their Antagonists," *Archives of Sexual Behavior,* 13, no. 5 (1985), 498.

9. Monica Schoelch-Krieger and R. J. Barfield, "Independence of Temporal Patterning of Male Mating Behavior from the Influence of Androgen during the Neonatal Period," *Physiology of Behavior,* 14 (1975), 251–55; G. Morali, L. Carillo, and C. Beyer, "Neonatal Androgen Influences Sexual Motivation but Not the Masculine Copulatory Motor Pattern in the Rat," *Physiology of Behavior,* 34 (1985), 267.

10. For a summary by authors who defend the validity of the theory, see Pieter van der Schoot and A. Kooy, "Current Topics in the Study of Sexual Behavior in Rats," in J. M. A. Sitsen, ed., *Handbook of Sexology,* vol. 6: *The Pharmacology and Endocrinology of Sexual Function* (Amsterdam: Elsevier, 1988), pp. 145–92.

11. Brian J. Whipp and Susan A. Ward, "Will Women Soon Outrun Men?" *Nature,* 355 (January 2, 1992), 25.

12. "Are Women Destined to Outpace Men?" *International Herald Tribune,* January 3, 1992.

13. We have to consider that this extrapolation and prediction of the records of women and men is valid only if the curve does not level off. We have no way of knowing a priori whether women hit some upper limit or, as have men, reach a point where their rate of improvement slows down so that it will not reach that of men.

14. Janet S. Hyde and M. C. Linn, "Gender Differences in Verbal Ability: A Meta-analysis," *Psychological Bulletin,* 104, no. 1 (1988), 53–69; Janet S. Hyde, E. Fennema, and S. J. Lamon, "Gender Differences in Mathematics Performance: A Meta-analysis," *Psychological Bulletin,* 107, no. 2 (1990), 139–55.

15. A female scientist is not necessarily a feminist. Female scientists usually do not appreciate being mentioned as women; the quality of their research is more important to them. Moreover, questions for research originating from feminist ideas are often qualified as not objective and thus not scientific. In many laboratories the ideology of the production of neutral, objective knowledge still prevails.

16. See Birke, *Women, Feminism and Biology,* esp. chap. 5.

17. Ibid., p. 104.

18. Ibid., esp. chap. 5.

19. Plan voor Positieve Aktie, Fakulteit Biologie, Universiteit van Amsterdam, September 1991.

20. Nelly Oudshoorn, *Beyond the Natural Body: An Archeology of the Origins of the Hormonal Body* (London: Routledge, 1994).

21. Sandra Harding and Merill B. Hintikka, eds., *Discovering Reality: Feminist Perspectives on Epistemology, Metaphysics, Methodology, and Philosophy of Science* (Dordrecht: Reidel, 1983).

22. Ruth Hubbard, "Have Only Men Evolved?" in Harding and Hintikka, eds., *Discovering Reality*.

23. Elizabeth Fischer criticized "natural selection," especially its presupposed effectiveness according to traditional biological views. She considers it excessively simplistic to suppose that all changes in an organism are advantageous to the organism or its species. Fischer mentions the change to erect walking in humans, which makes childbirth more difficult. Efficiency presupposes appropriateness, and it is questionable whether that is nature's aim. See Elizabeth Fischer, *Woman's Creation* (New York: Anchor, 1979). Sarah Blaffer Hrdy (and many others) criticized "sexual selection" and "competition": Sarah Blaffer Hrdy, *The Woman That Never Evolved* (Cambridge: Harvard University Press, 1983).

24. Elaine Morgan, *De vrouw onze voorvader* (Amsterdam: Elsevier, 1972); Evelyn Reed, *Women's Evolution* (New York: Pathfinders, 1975).

25. Bleier, *Science and Gender*, esp. chap. 5. For an overview of authors who published on this subject, see Berry Ramakers and Sylvia Borg, *Wat deed de vrouw terwijl de man op jacht was?* (Women's Studies Biology, University of Amsterdam, 1985).

26. Bleier, *Science and Gender*, p. 117.

27. In the Netherlands, a popularized version of this study was published at the request of a publisher of popular scientific books; see Marianne van den Wijngaard, *Het eeuwenoude misverstand. De invloed van de hersenen op het gedrag van mannen en vrouwen* (Bloemendaal: Aramith, 1993). Its publication drew extensive media coverage.

28. Annemarie Mol, "Sekse, rijkdom en bloedarmoede: Over lokaliseren als strategie," *Tijdschrift voor Vrouwenstudies*, 11, no. 42 (1990), 142–58. Mol analyzed the social and material conditions under which the diagnosis "anemia" can "work" in medical practice and how this affects women's lives.

Alcoff, Linda. "Cultural Feminism Versus Post-Structuralism: The Identity Crisis in Feminist Theory," *Signs: Journal of Women in Culture and Society,* 13, no. 31 (1988), 405–36.

Anderson, C. O., M. X. Zarrow, and V. H. Denenberg. "Maternal Behavior in the Rabbit: Effects of Androgen Treatment during Gestation upon the Nest-Building Behaviors of the Mother and Her Offspring," *Hormones and Behavior,* 1 (1970), 337–45.

Anonymous. "Be Open and Honest with Sufferers," *British Medical Journal,* 306 (April 16, 1994), 1041–42.

Anonymous. "Once a Dark Secret," *British Medical Journal,* 305 (February 19, 1994), 542.

Arnold, Arthur P., and Roger A. Gorski. "Gonadal Steroid Induction of Structural Sex Differences in the Central Nervous System," *Annual Review of Neuroscience,* 7 (1984), 413–42.

Beach, Frank A. "Behavioral Endocrinology: An Emerging Discipline," *American Scientist,* 63 (1975), 178–87.

———. "Historical Origins of Modern Research on Hormones and Behavior," *Hormones and Behavior,* 15 (1981), 325–76.

———. "Hormonal Control of Sex-Related Behavior," in Frank A. Beach, ed., *Human Sexuality in Four Perspectives.* Baltimore: Johns Hopkins University Press, 1977.

———. "Hormonal Factors Controlling the Differentiation, Development and Display of Copulatory Behaviors in the Ramstergig (!) and Related Species," pp. 249–96 in Ethel Tobach, Lester R. Aronson, and Evelyn Shaw, eds., *The Biopsychology of Development.* New York: Academic, 1971.

———. "Sexual Attractivity, Proceptivity and Receptivity in Female Mammals," *Hormones and Behavior,* 7 (1976), 105–38.

Beauvoir, Simone de. *The Second Sex,* trans. H. M. Parshley. New York: Knopf, 1953.

Bell, Susan E. "Changing Ideas: The Medicalization of Menopause," *Social Science and Medicine,* 24 (1987), 535–42.

———. "A New Model of Medical Technology Development: A Case Study of DES," *Research in the Sociology of Health Care,* 4 (1986), 1–33.

Bem, Sandra L. "The Measurement of Psychological Androgyny," *Journal of Consulting and Clinical Psychology,* 42 (1972), 155–62.

Benbow, Camilla, and Julian Stanley. "Sex Differences in Mathematical Ability: Fact or Artefact?" *Science,* 210 (1980), 1262–64.

Benno, R., and T. Williams. "Evidence for Intracellular Localization of Alpha-fetoprotein in the Developing Rat Brain," *Brain Research,* 142 (1978), 182–86.

Bermant, Gordon. "Response Latencies of Female Rats during Sexual Intercourse," *Science,* 133 (1961), 1771–73.

Birke, Lynda. *Women, Feminism and Biology: The Feminist Challenge.* Brighton: Harvester, 1986.

Bleier, Ruth. *Science and Gender: A Critique of Biology and Its Theories on Women.* New York: Pergamon, 1984.

Boers, Chris. *Wetenschap, techniek en samenleving: Bouwstenen voor een kritische wetenschapstheorie.* Meppel: Boom, 1981.

Brodie, H. K. H., et al. "Plasma Testosterone Levels in Heterosexual and Homosexual Men," *New England Journal of Medicine,* 289 (1973), 1236–38.

Brouns, Margo. *Veertien jaar vrouwenstudies in Nederland.* 's Gravenhage: Ministerie van Onderwijs en Wetenschappen, 1988.

Brown-Grant, K., A. Munck, F. Naftolin, and M. R. Sherwood. "The Effects of the Administration of Testosterone Propionate Alone or with Phenobarbiturone and of Testosterone Metabolites to Neonatal Female Rats," *Hormones and Behavior,* 2 (1971), 173–82.

Browne, F. *Postgraduate Obstetrics and Gynecology.* London Butterworths, 1950.

Buffery, A. W. H., and J. A. Gray. "Sex Differences in the Development of Spatial and Linguistic Skills," in C. Onsted and D. C. Taylor, eds., *Gender Differences: Their Onthogeny and Significance.* London: Churchill Livingstone, 1975.

Burt, Ronald S. *Toward a Structural Theory of Action.* New York: Academic, 1982.

Butler, Judith. *Gender Trouble: Feminism and the Subversion of Identity.* New York: Routledge, 1990.

Calhoun, J. B. *The Ecology and Sociology of the Norway Rat.* Washington, D.C.: U.S. Government Printing Office, 1962.

Clarke, Adele E. "Embryology and the Rise of American Reproductive Sciences," pp. 107–32 in *The American Expansion of Biology,* ed. Keith Benson, Ronald Raigner, and Jane Maienschein. New Brunswick: Rutgers University Press, 1993.

Constantinople, Anne. "Masculinity-Femininity: An Exception to a Famous Dictum?" *Psychological Bulletin,* 80, no. 5 (1973), 389–407.

Dawkins, Richard. *The Selfish Gene.* Oxford, Oxford University Press, 1976.

de Lauretis, Teresa, Luce Irigaray, and Gayatri Spivak. Contributions in "The Essential Difference: Another Look at Essentialism," *Differences: A Journal of Feminist Cultural Studies,* 1 (1989).

Dis, Huib van, and Nanne E. v.d. Poll. "Sexual Differentiation of Behavior in Rats," *Progress in Brain Research,* 41 (1974), 321–31.

Dixon, A. F., G. J. Everitt, J. Herbert, S. W. Rugman, and D. M. Scruton. "Hormonal and Other Determinants of Sexual Attractiveness and Receptivity in Rhesus and Talapoin Monkeys," pp. 41, 42 in IVth International Congress on Primatology, 1973, vol. 2: *Primate Reproductive Behavior.* Basel: Karger, 1974.

Doerr, Peter, et al. "Further Studies on Sex Hormones in Male Homosexuals," *Archives of General Psychiatry,* 33 (1976), 611–14.

———. "Plasma Testosterone, Estradiol and Semen Analysis in Male Homosexuals," *Archives of General Psychiatry,* 29 (1973), 829–33.

Döhler, Klaus D. "Is Female Sexual Differentiation Hormone-mediated?" *Trends in Neurosciences,* 1 (1978), 138–40.

Döhler, Klaus D., and W. Wuttke. "Changes with Age in Levels of Serum

Gonadotropins, Prolactin and Gonadal Steroids in Prepubertal Male and Female Rats," *Endocrinology*, 97 (1975), 898–907.

Dörner, G., et al. "Hormonal Induction and Prevention of Female Homosexuality," *Archives of Sexual Behavior*, 4 (1979), 1–9.

Dörner, Günther, and G. Hinz. "Induction and Prevention of Male Homosexuality by Androgen," *Journal of Endocrinology*, 40 (1968), 387–88.

Doty, Richard L. "A Cry for the Liberation of the Female Rodent: Courtship and Copulation in Rodentia," *Psychological Bulletin*, 31 (1974), 159–73.

Durden-Smith, John, and Diana De Simone. *Sex and the Brain*. London: Pan, 1983.

Echols, Alice. "The New Feminism of Yin and Yang," in Ann Snitow, Christine Stansell, and Sharon Thompson, eds., *Powers of Desire: The Politics of Sexuality*. New York: Monthly Review Press, 1983.

Ehrhardt, Anke A. "Gender Differences: A Biosocial Perspective," pp. 37–59 in Richard A. Dienstbier and Theo B. Sonderegger, eds., *Current Theory and Research in Motivation*, vol. 32. Lincoln: University of Nebraska Press, 1985.

Ehrhardt, Anke A., and Heino F. L. Meyer-Bahlburg. "Effects of Prenatal Sex Hormones on Gender-related Behavior," *Science*, 211 (1981), 1312–18.

Ehrhardt, Anke A., G. C. Grisanti, and H. F. L. Meyer-Bahlburg. "Prenatal Exposure to Medroxyprogesterone Acetate (MPA) in Girls," *Psychoneuroendocrinology*, 2 (1977), 391–98.

Ehrhardt, Anke A., S. E. Ince, and Heino F. L. Meyer-Bahlburg. "Career Aspiration and Gender Role Development in Young Girls," *Archives of Sexual Behavior*, 10, no. 3 (1981), 281–99.

Ehrhardt, Anke A., Heino F. L. Meyer-Bahlburg, Laura R. Rosen, Judith F. Feldman, Norma P. Veridiano, I. Zimmerman, and Bruce S. McEwen. "Sexual Orientation after Prenatal Exposure to Exogenous Estrogen," *Archives of Sexual Behavior*, 14, no. 1 (1985), 57–76.

Emery, Donna, and R. L. Moss. "Lesions Confined to the Ventromedial Hypothalamus Decrease the Frequency of Coital Contacts in Female Rats," *Hormones and Behavior*, 18 (1984), 313–29.

Epstein, Julia. *Altered Conditions: Disease, Medicine and Storytelling*. New York: Routledge, 1995.

———. "Either/Or–Neither/Both: Sexual Ambiguity and the Ideology of Gender," *Genders*, 7 (1990), 99–142.

Erskine, Mary S. "Solicitation Behavior in the Estrous Female Rat: A Review," *Hormones and Behavior*, 23 (1989), 473–502.

Everitt, B. J., J. Herbert, and J. D. Hamer. "Sexual Receptivity of Bilaterally Adrenalectomized Female Rhesus Monkeys," *Physiology of Behavior*, 8 (1971), 409–15.

Fausto-Sterling, Anne. "The Five Sexes: Why Male and Female Are Not Enough," *The Sciences* (March-April 1993), 20–24.

———. "Life in the XY Corral," *Women's Studies International Forum*, 12, no. 3 (1989), 319–31.

———. *Myths of Gender: Biological Theories of Women and Men*. New York: Basic, 1985.

———. "Society Writes Biology, Biology Constructs Gender," *Daedalus*, 116 (1987), 61–76.

Fee, Elizabeth. "Nineteenth Century Craniology: The Study of the Female Skull," *Bulletin of the History of Medicine,* 53 (1979), 415–33.

Fischer, Elizabeth. *Woman's Creation.* New York: Anchor, 1979.

Foucault, Michel. *Herculine Barbin, dite Alexina B. presenté par Michel Foucault.* Paris: Gallimard, 1978. Dutch translation includes an introduction by Foucault: Herculine Barbin, *Mijn herinneringen.* Amsterdam: Arbeiderspers, 1982.

———. *Histoire de la sexualité.* 1. *La volonté de savoir.* Paris: Gallimard, 1976. English translation: *The History of Sexuality.* New York: Vintage, 1980.

Freeman, D. *Mead and Samoa: The Making and Unmaking of an Anthropological Myth.* Cambridge: Harvard University Press, 1983.

Fried, Barbara. "Boys Will Be Boys Will Be Boys: The Language of Sex and Gender," in Ruth Hubbard, M. S. Henifin, and B. Fried, eds., *Women Look at Biology Looking at Women.* Cambridge: Schenkman, 1979.

———. "What Is a Woman?" in Ruth Hubbard, Mary Sue Henifin, and Barbara Fried, *Women Look at Biology Looking at Women.* Cambridge: Schenkman, 1978.

Geschwind, Norman. "Biological Foundations of Cerebral Dominance," *Trends in Neurosciences,* 6, no. 9 (1983), 354–56.

Geschwind, Norman, and Albert Galaburda. "Cerebral Lateralization," *Archives of Neurology,* 42 (1985), 428–59.

Goodman, L. S., and A. Gilman. *The Pharmacological Basis of Therapeutics.* 5th ed. New York: Macmillan, 1975.

Goodman, Raymond E. "Biology of Sexuality: Inborn Determinants of Human Sexual Response," *British Journal of Psychiatry,* 143 (1983), 216–55.

Gorski, Roger A. "Gonadal Hormones and the Perinatal Development of Neuroendocrine Function," in L. Martini and W. F. Ganong, eds., *Frontiers in Neuroendocrinology.* New York: Oxford University Press, 1971.

———. "Modification of Ovulatory Mechanisms by Postnatal Administration of Estrogen to the Rat," *American Journal of Physiology,* 205 (1963), 842–44.

———. "The Neuroendocrinology of Reproduction. An Overview," *Biology of Reproduction,* 20 (1979), 111–27.

Goy, Robert W. "William Caldwell Young, 1899–1965," pp. 5–11 in J. Meites, B. T. Donovan, and S. McCann, eds., *Pioneers in Neuroendocrinology.* New York: Plenum, 1975.

Goy, Robert, and Bruce McEwen. *Sexual Differentiation of the Brain: Based on a Work Session of the Neurosciences Program.* Cambridge: MIT Press, 1980.

Greer, Germaine. *The Female Eunuch.* London: MacGibbon and Kee, 1970.

Haraway, Donna. "The Contest for Primate Nature: Daughters of Man the Hunter in the Field, 1960–1980," pp. 175–207 in M. Kann, ed., *The Future of American Democracy.* Philadelphia: Temple University Press, 1983.

———. "Situated Knowledges: The Science Question in Feminism and the Privilege of Partial Perspective," *Feminist Studies,* 14, no. 3 (1988), 575–99.

Harding, Sandra. "How the Women's Movement Benefits Science: Two Views," *Women's Studies International Forum,* 12, no. 3 (1989), 271–83.

———. *The Science Question in Feminism.* Ithaca: Cornell University Press, 1986.

Harding, Sandra, and Merill B. Hintikka, eds. *Discovering Reality. Feminist Perspectives on Epistemology, Metaphysics, Methodology, and Philosophy of Science*. Dordrecht: Reidel, 1983.

Herdt, G. H., and J. Davidson. "The Sambia 'Turnim-man': Sociocultural and Clinical Aspects of Gender Formation in Male Pseudohermaphrodites with 5 Alpha Reductase Deficiency in Papua New Guinea," *Archives of Sexual Behavior*, 17, no. 1 (1988), 33.

Hines, Melissa. "Prenatal Diethylstilbesterol (DES) Exposure, Human Sexually Dimorphic Behavior and Cerebral Lateralization" (Ph.D. dissertation, University of California, Los Angeles, 1981), *Dissertation Abstracts International*, 42 (1981), 423B.

———. "Prenatal Gonadal Hormones and Sex Differences in Human Behavior," *Psychological Bulletin*, 92, no. 1 (1982), 56–80.

Hirschauer, Stefan. "The Manufacture of Bodies in Surgery," *Social Studies of Science*, 21 (1991), 279–319.

Hrdy, Sarah Blaffer. *The Woman That Never Evolved*. Cambridge: Harvard University Press, 1983.

Hubbard, Ruth. "Have Only Men Evolved," in S. Harding and M. B. Hintikka, eds., *Discovering Reality: Feminist Perspectives on Epistemology, Metaphysics, Methodology and Philosophy of Science*. Dordrecht: Reidel, 1983.

———. *The Politics of Women's Biology*. New Brunswick: Rutgers University Press, 1990.

Hyde, Janet S., and M. C. Linn. "Gender Differences in Verbal Ability: A Meta-analysis," *Psychological Bulletin*, 104, no. 1 (1988), 53–69.

Hyde, Janet S., E. Fennema, and S. J. Lamon. "Gender Differences in Mathematics Performance: A Meta-analysis," *Psychological Bulletin*, 107, no. 2 (1990), 139–55.

Jagentowicz Mill, Patricia. *Women, Nature, and Psyche*. New Haven: Yale University Press, 1987.

Jonge, Francien H. de. "Sexual and Aggressive Behavior in Female Rats: Psychological and Endocrine Factors" (Ph.D. thesis, University of Amsterdam, 1986).

Jordanova, Ludmilla. *Sexual Visions: Images of Gender in Science and Medicine between the Eighteenth and Twentieth Centuries*. Madison: University of Wisconsin Press, 1989.

Jost, A. "Hormonal Influences in the Development of the Fetus," *Cold Spring Harbor Symposium on Quantitative Biology*, 19 (1954), 3–9.

———. "Hormonal Influences in the Development of the Fetus," *Cold Spring Harbor Symposium on Quantitative Biology*, 1964), 167–81.

Keller, Evelyn Fox. *A Feeling for the Organism: The Life and Work of Barbara McClintock*. New York: Freeman, 1983.

———. *Reflections on Gender and Science*. New Haven: Yale University Press, 1985.

Kesler Unger, Rhoda. "Through the Looking Glass: No Wonderland Yet! (The Reciprocal Relationship between Methodology and Models of Reality)," *Psychology of Women Quarterly*, 8, no. 1 (1983), 9–33.

Kessler, S., and W. McKenna. "Toward a Theory of Gender," in *Gender, an Ethnomethodological Approach*. New York: Wiley, 1978.

Kloos, P. "De aanval op Margareth Mead." *Intermediair,* 19, no. 28, July 15, 1983.

———. *Door het oog van de anthropoloog. Botsende visiesbij heronderzoek.* Muiderberg: Coutinho, 1988.

Kuhn, Thomas. *The Structure of Scientific Revolutions.* Chicago: University of Chicago Press, 1970.

Lacoste-Utamsing, Christine de, and Ralph Holloway. "Sexual Dimorphism in the Human Corpus Callosum," *Science,* 216 (1982), 1431–32.

Laqueur, Thomas. *Making Sex: Body and Gender from the Greeks to Freud.* Cambridge: Harvard University Press, 1990.

Latour, Bruno. "Give Me a Laboratory and I Will Raise the World," pp. 141–71 in Karin Knorr and Michael Mulkay, eds., *Science Observed: Perspectives on the Social Studies of Science.* London: Sage, 1983.

———. *Science in Action: How to Follow Scientists and Engineers through Society.* Milton Keynes: Open University Press, 1987.

Latour, Bruno, and Steve Woolgar. *Laboratory Life: The Social Construction of Scientific Facts.* Beverly Hills: Sage, 1979.

Law, John. "Technology, Closure and Heterogeneous Engineering: The Case of the Portuguese Expansion," in Wiebe Bijker, Trevor Pinch, and Thomas P. Hughes eds., *The Social Construction of Technological Systems.* Cambridge: MIT Press, 1987.

Leavitt, Judith Walzer, and Linda Gordon. "A Decade of Feminist Critiques in the Natural Sciences: An Address by Ruth Bleier," *Signs: Journal of Women in Culture and Society,* 14, no. 1 (1988), 182–96.

Lewontin, Richard, Steven Rose, and Leon Kamin. *Not in Our Genes: Biology, Ideology and Human Nature.* New York: Pantheon, 1984.

Long Hall, Diana. "Biology, Sex Hormones and Sexism in the 1920s," in Carol C. Gould and Marx W. Wartofsky, eds., *Women and Philosophy.* New York: Putnam, 1976.

Longino, Helen E. *Science as Social Knowledge: Values and Objectivity in Scientific Inquiry.* Princeton: Princeton University Press, 1990.

Longino, Helen, and Ruth Doel. "Body, Bias, and Behavior: A Comparative Analysis of Reasoning in Two Areas of Biological Science," *Signs: Journal of Women in Culture and Society,* 9, no. 2 (1983), 207–27.

Maccoby, Eleanor, and Carol Jacklin. *The Psychology of Sex Differences.* Stanford: Stanford University Press, 1974.

Madlafousek, Jaroslav, and Zdenek Hlinak. "Analysis of Factors Determining the Appetitive and Aversive Phase of Sexual Behavior in the Female Rat," *Physiologica Bohemoslovenica,* 21 (1972), 416–17.

———. "The Dependence of Sexual Behavior of Inexperienced Males on the Precopulatory Behavior of Females in Albino Rat," *Physiologica Bohemoslovenica,* 21 (1972), 83–84.

——— "Importance of Female's Precopulatory Behaviour for the Primary Initiation of Male's Copulatory Behavior in the Laboratory Rat," *Behaviour,* 86 (1983), 237–49.

———. "Sexual Behavior of the Female Laboratory Rat: Inventory, Patterning, and Measurement," *Behaviour* 63 (1977), 129–74.

McClintock, Martha K., J. J. Anisko, and N. J. Adler. "The Role of the Female during Copulation in Wild and Domestic Norway Rats *(Rattus norvegicus),*" *Behaviour,* 67 (1982), 67–96.

McCrea, Frances B., and Gerald E. Markle. "The Estrogen Replacement Controversy in the USA and UK: Different Answers to the Same Question?" *Social Studies of Science,* 14 (1984), 1–26.

McDonald, P., C. Beyer, F. Newton, B. Brien, R. Bake, H. S. Tan, C. Sampson, P. Kitching, R. Greenhill, and D. Pritchard. "Failure of 5a-Dihydrotestosterone to Initiate Sexual Behaviour in the Castrated Male Rat," *Nature,* 227 (1970), 964–65.

McEwen, Bruce. "Gonadal Steroid Receptors in Neuroendocrine Tissues," pp. 353–400 in B. O'Malley and I. Birnbaumer, eds., *Hormone Receptors,* vol. 1: *Steroid Hormones.* New York: Academic, 1978.

McEwen, Bruce, I. Lieberburg, C. Chaptal, and L. C. Krey. "Role of Fetoneonatal Estrogen Binding Proteins in the Association of Estrogens with Neonatal Brain Cell Nuclear Receptors," *Brain Research,* 96 (1975), 400–406.

Mead, Margaret. *Coming of Age.* New York: Mentor, 1949.

———. *Coming of Age in Samoa.* New York: Morrow, 1928.

———. *Male and Female: A Study of the Sexes in a Changing World.* New York: Morrow, 1949.

———. *Sex and Temperament in Three Primitive Societies.* New York: Morrow, 1935.

Meyer, M. Mellcow. "Tumors of Dysgenetic Gonads in Intersexes: Case Reports and Discussion Regarding Their Place in Gonadal Oncology," *Bulletin of the New York Academy of Medicine,* 42, no. 3 (1966).

Meyer-Bahlburg, Heino F. L. "Psychoendocrine Research on Sexual Orientation: Current Status and Future Options," *Progress in Brain Research,* 61 (1984), 375–98.

Meyer-Bahlburg, Heino F. L., A. A. Ehrhardt, L. R. Rosen, J. F. Feldman, N. P. Veridiano, I. Zimmerman, and B. S. McEwen. "Psychosexual Milestones in Women Prenatally Exposed to Diethylbestrol," *Hormones and Behavior,* 18 (1984), 359–66.

Meyerson, B. J., and L. H. Lindström. "Sexual Motivation in the Female Rat: A Methodological Study Applied to the Investigation of the Effects of Estradiol-benzoate," *Acta Physiologica Scandinavica,* Suppl. 389 (1973), 1–80.

Mitchell, Juliet. "On Freud and the Distinction between the Sexes," in Jean Strouse, ed., *Women and Analysis, Dialogues on Psychoanalytic Views of Femininity.* New York: Dell, 1974.

Moir, Anne, and David Jessel. *BrainSex: The REAL Difference between MEN and WOMEN.* London: Michael Joseph, 1989.

Mol, Annemarie. "Baarmoeders, pigment en pyramiden. Over de vraag of anti-racisten en feministen er goed aan doen 'de biologie' haar plaats te wijzen," *Tijdschrift voor vrouwenstudies,* 35 (1988), 276–90.

———. "Sekse, rijkdom en bloedarmoede. Over loka liseren als strategie," *Tijdschrift voor Vrouwenstudies,* 11, no. 42 (1990), 142–58.

Money, John. *Love and Love Sickness: The Science of Sex, Gender Difference, and Pair-Bonding.* Baltimore: Johns Hopkins University Press, 1980.

————. "Sex Hormones and Other Variables in Human Eroticism," pp. 1383–1400 in W. C. Young, ed., *Sex and Internal Secretions.* 3rd ed. Baltimore: Williams and Wilkins, 1961.

Money, John, and Anke A. Ehrhardt. *Man and Woman, Boy and Girl: Differentiation and Dimorphism of Gender Identity from Conception to Maturity.* Baltimore: Johns Hopkins University Press, 1972.

Money, John, and A. J. Russo. "Homosexual Outcome of Discordant Gender Identity/Role in Childhood: Longitudinal Follow-up," *Journal of Pediatric Psychology,* 4 (1979), 29–41.

Money, John, Joan G. Hampson, and John L. Hampson. "An Examination of Some Basic Sexual Concepts: The Evidence of Human Hermaphroditism," *Bulletin Johns Hopkins Hospital,* 97 (1955), 301–19.

Moore, Celia. "Another Psychobiological View of Sexual Differentiation," *Developmental Review,* 5 (1985), 18–55.

————. "Maternal Behavior of Rats is Affected by Hormonal Condition of Pups," *Journal of Comparative and Physiological Psychology,* 96, no. 1 (1982), 123–29.

————. "Maternal Contributions to the Development of Masculine Sexual Behavior in Laboratory Rats," *Developmental Psychobiology,* 17 (1984), 347–56.

Moore, C. R. "On the Physiological Properties of the Gonads as Controllers of Somatic and Psychical Characteristics," *Journal of Experimental Zoology,* 28 (1919), 137.

Morali, G., L. Carillo, and C. Beyer. "Neonatal Androgen Influences Sexual Motivation but Not the Masculine Copulatory Motor Pattern in the Rat," *Physiology of Behavior,* 34 (1985), 267.

Morgan, Elaine. *The Descent of Woman.* London: Souvenir, 1972.

Naftolin, F. "Understanding the Bases of Sex Differences," *Science,* 211 (1981), 1263–64.

Naftolin, F., K. J. Ryan, and Z. Petro. "Aromatization of Androstenedione by the Anterior Hypothalamus of Adult Male and Female Rats," *Endocrinology,* 90 (1972), 295–98.

————. "Aromatization of Androstenedione by Limbic System Tissue from Human Fetuses," *Journal of Endocrinology,* 51 (1971), 795–96.

Oakley, Ann. *Subject Woman.* New York: Pantheon, 1981.

Ojeda, S. R., P. S. Kalra, and S. M. McCann. "Further Studies on the Maturation of the Estrogen Negative Feedback on Gonadotropin Release in the Female Rat," *Neuroendocrinology,* 18 (1975), 242–55.

Oudshoorn, Nelly. *Beyond the Natural Body: An Archeology of Sex Hormones.* London: Routledge, 1994.

————. "Endocrinologists and the Conceptualization of Sex, 1920–1940," *Journal of the History of Biology,* 23 (1990), 163–86.

Oudshoorn, Nelly, and Marianne van den Wijngaard. "Dualism in Biology: The Case of Sex-hormones," *Women's Studies International Forum,* 14, no. 5 (1991), 459–71.

Phoenix, Charles H., Roger W. Goy, Arnold A. Gerall, and William C. Young.

"Organization Action of Testosterone Propionate on the Tissues Mediating Mating Behaviors in the Female Guinea Pig," *Endocrinology,* 65 (1959), 369–82.

Pomata, Gianna. "De geschiedenis van vrouwen: een kwestie van grenzen," *Socialistisch Feministische Teksten,* 10 (1987), 61–113.

Price, Dorothy. "Feedback Control of Gonadal and Hypophyseal Hormones: Evolution of the Concept," in Joseph Meites, Bernal T. Donovan, Samuel M. McCann, eds., *Pioneers in Neuroendocrinology.* New York: Plenum, 1975.

Quadagno, David M., Robert Briscoe, and Jill. S. Quadagno. "Effects of Perinatal Gonadal Hormones on Selected Nonsexual Behavior Patterns: A Critical Assessment of the Nonhuman and Human Literature," *Psychological Bulletin,* 84, no. 1 (1977), 62–80.

Reed, Evelyn. *Women's Evolution.* New York: Pathfinders, 1975.

Reinisch, June M. "Effects of Prenatal Hormone Exposure on Physical and Psychological Development in Humans and Animals: With a Note on the State of the Field," in Edward J. Sachar, ed., *Hormones, Behavior, and Psychopathology.* New York: Raven, 1976.

———. "Prenatal Exposure of Human Foetuses to Synthetic Progestin and Oestrogen Affects Personality," *Nature,* 266 (1977), 561–62.

———. "Prenatal Exposure to Synthetic Progestins Increases Potential for Aggression in Humans," *Science,* 211 (1981), 1171–73.

Reinisch, June M., and W. G. Karow. "Prenatal Exposure to Synthetic Progestins and Estrogens: Effects on Human Development," *Archives of Sexual Behavior,* 6 (1977), 257–88.

Resko, John, J. Ploem, and H. Stadelman. "Estrogens in Fetal and Maternal Plasma of the Rhesus Monkey," *Endocrinology,* 97 (1975), 425–30.

Rose, Hilary, and Steven Rose. "On Oppositions to Reductionism," pp. 50–59 in Dialectics of Biology Group, ed., *Against Biological Determinism.* London: Allison and Busby, 1982.

Sahlins, M. *The Use and Abuse of Biology.* London, 1977.

Sanday, P. Reeves. "Margaret Mead's View on Sex Roles in Her Own and Other Societies," *American Anthropologist,* 82, no. 2 (1980), 340–48.

Sayers, Janet. *Biological Politics, Feminist and Anti-Feminist Perspectives.* London: Tavistock, 1982.

Schiebinger, Londa. "Skeletons in the Closet: The First Illustrations of the Female Skeleton in the 19th-century Anatomy," *Representations,* 14 (1986), 42–83.

Schoelch-Krieger, Monica, and R. J. Barfield. "Independence of Temporal Patterning of Male Mating Behavior from the Influence of Androgen during the Neonatal Period," *Physiology of Behavior,* 14 (1975), 251–55.

Schoot, Pieter van der, and A. Kooy. "Current Topics in the Study of Sexual Behavior in Rats," pp. 145–92 in J. M. A. Sitsen, ed., *Handbook of Sexology,* vol. 6: *The Pharmacology and Endocrinology of Sexual Function.* Amsterdam: Elsevier, 1988.

Seters, A. P. van, and A. K. Slob. "Mutually Gratifying Heterosexual Relationship with Micropenis of Husband," *Journal of Sex and Marital Therapy,* 14 (1988), 97–104.

Shapiro, Bernard. "A Paradox in Development: Masculinization of the Brain without Receptors," *Progress in Clinical and Biological Research (US)*, 171 (1985), 151–73.

Slaughter, Mary, Richard Wilen, Kenneth J. Ryan, and Frederic Naftolin. "The Effects of Low Dose Diethylstilbesterol Administration in Neonatal Female Rats," *Journal of Steroid Biochemistry*, 8 (1977), 621–23.

Slijper, Froukje M. E. "Androgens and Gender Role Behavior in Girls with Congenital Adrenal Hyperplasia (CAH)," *Progress in Brain Research*, 61 (1984), 417–23.

———. *Gender Role Behavior in Girls with Congenital Adrenal Hyperplasia.* (Ph.D. thesis, Department of Child Psychiatry, Erasmus University, Rotterdam).

Södersten, Per. "Increased Mounting Behavior in the Female Rat Following a Single Neonatal Injection of Testosterone Propionate," *Hormones and Behavior*, 4 (1973), 1–17.

Södersten, Per, and J. A. Gustafsson. "A Way in Which Estradiol Might Play a Role in the Sexual Behavior of Male Rats," *Hormones and Behavior*, 14 (1980), 271–74.

Spence, Janet T., Robert Helmreich, and Joy Stapp. "Ratings of Self and Peers on Sex Role Attributes and Their Relation to Self-Esteem and Conceptions of Masculinity and Femininity," *Journal of Personality and Social Psychology*, 32, no. 1 (1975), 29–39.

Star, Susan L. "Scientific Work and Uncertainty," *Social Studies of Science*, 15 (1985), 391–427.

———. "Simplification in Scientific Work: An Example from Neuro-endocrine Research," *Social Studies of Science*, 13 (1983), 205–208.

———. "The Sociology of the Invisible: The Primacy of Work in the Writings of Anselm Strauss," in David R. Maines, ed., *Social Organization and Social Process: Essays in Honor of Anselm Strauss.* New York: Aldine de Gruyter, 1991.

Steinach, E. "Feminisierung von Männchen und Masculinisierung von Weibchen," *Zentralblatt für Physiologie*, 27 (1913).

Swaab, D. F., and M. A. Hofman. "Sexual Differentiation of the Human Brain: A Historical Perspective," *Progress in Brain Research*, 61 (1984), 361–75.

Swaab, Dick, and E. Fliers. "A Sexually Dimorphic Nucleus in the Human Brain," *Science*, 228 (1985), 1112–16.

Tiefer, Leonore. "The Context and Consequences of Contemporary Sex Research: A Feminist Perspective," pp. 363–85 in T. E. McGill, D. A. Dewsbury, and B. D. Sachs, eds., *Sex and Behavior: Status and Prospectus.* New York: Plenum, 1978.

———. "Feminism and Sex Research: Ten Years' Reminiscences and Appraisal," pp. 87–101 in Joan C. Chrisler and Doris Howard, eds., *New Directions in Feminist Psychology.* New York: Springer, 1992.

———. "In Memoriam, Frank A. Beach," *Hormones and Behavior*, 22 (1988), 419–43.

Trivers, Robert. "Parental Investment and Sexual Selection," in B. Campbell, ed., *Sexual Selection and the Descent of Man.* Chicago: Aldine, 1972.

Trumbach, Randolph. "London Sodomites: Homosexual Behavior and Western Culture in the Eighteenth Century," *Journal of Social History,* 11 (1977), 1–33.

Urbach, P. "Progress and Degeneration in the "IQ debate," *British Journal of the Philosophy of Science,* 25 (1974), 99–36 and 235–59.

Vetterling-Braggin, Mary, ed. *"Femininity," "Masculinity" and "Androgyny": A Modern Philosophical Discussion.* Totowa, N.J.: Littlefield Adams, 1982.

Whalen, Richard E. "Hormone-induced Changes in the Organization of Sexual Behavior in the Male Rat," *Journal of Comparative Physiological Psychology,* 57 (1964), 175–82.

———. "Multiple Actions of Steroids and Their Antagonists," *Archives of Sexual Behavior,* 13, no. 5 (1985), 498–502.

———. "Sexual Differentiation: Models, Methods and Mechanisms," in R. C. Friedman, R. M. Richart, R. L. Van de Wiele, eds., *Sex Differences in Behavior.* New York: Krüger, 1974.

Whalen, Richard E., and Anne M. Etgen. "Masculinization and Defeminization Induced in Female Hamsters by Neonatal Treatment with Estradiol Benzoate and RU-2858," *Hormones and Behavior,* 10 (1978), 170–77.

Whalen, Richard E., and R. D. Nadler. "Modification of Spontaneous and Hormone Induced Sexual Behavior by Estrogen Administered to Neonatal Female Rats," *Journal of Comparative Physiological Psychology,* 60 (1965).

———. "Suppression of the Development of Female Mating Behavior by Estrogen Administered in Infancy," *Science,* 141 (1963), 273–74.

Whalen, Richard E., and Robert W. Goy. "In Memoriam, Frank A. Beach," *Hormones and Behavior,* 22 (1988), 419–43.

Whipp, Brian J., and Susan A. Ward. "Will Women Soon Outrun Men?" *Nature,* 355 (January 2, 1992), 25.

Whitley, R. "The Establishment and Structure of the Sciences as Reputational Organizations," in N. Elias, H. Maihns, and R. Whitley, eds., *Scientific Establishments and Hierarchies, Sociology of the Sciences Yearbook.* Dordrecht: Reidel, 1982.

Wijngaard, Marianne van den. *Het eeuwenoude misverstand. De invloed van de hersenen op het gedrag van mannen en vrouwen.* Bloemendaal: Aramith, 1993.

———. "The Liberation of the Female Rodent," in Lynda Birke and Ruth Hubbard, eds., *Reinventing Biology.* Bloomington: Indiana University Press, 1995.

Wilson, E. O. *On Human Nature.* Cambridge: Harvard University Press, 1978.

———. *Sociobiology: The New Synthesis.* Cambridge: Belknap, 1975.

Yalom, Irvin, Richard Green, and Norman Fisk. "Prenatal Exposure to Female Hormones: Effect on Psychosexual Development in Boys," *Archives of General Psychiatry,* 28 (1973), 554–62.

Young, William C., Robert W. Goy, Charles H. Phoenix. "Hormones and Sexual Behavior: Broad Relationships Exist between the Gonadal Hormones and Behavior," *Science,* 143 (1964), 212–18.

MARIANNE VAN DEN WIJNGAARD is a biologist who developed courses in Women's Studies in the Department of Biology at the University of Amsterdam, The Netherlands. She has written many articles in both Dutch and English on her research on gender and biology. In the Netherlands a popular version of this book drew extensive media coverage.